Crying for Our Elders

Crying for Our Elders

African Orphanhood in the Age of HIV and AIDS

KRISTEN E. CHENEY

The University of Chicago Press
Chicago and London

The University of Chicago Press, Chicago 60637
The University of Chicago Press, Ltd., London
© 2017 by The University of Chicago
Published 2017.
Printed in the United States of America

27 26 25 24 23 22 21 20 19 18   2 3 4 5 6

ISBN-13: 978-0-226-43740-8 (cloth)
ISBN-13: 978-0-226-43754-5 (paper)
ISBN-13: 978-0-226-43768-2 (e-book)
DOI: 10.7208/CHICAGO/9780226437682.001.0001

Library of Congress Cataloging-in-Publication Data
Names: Cheney, Kristen E., author.
Title: Crying for our elders : African orphanhood in the age of HIV and AIDS / Kristen E. Cheney.
Description: Chicago ; London : The University of Chicago Press, 2017. | Includes bibliographical references and index.
Identifiers: LCCN 2016029264 | ISBN 9780226437408 (cloth : alk. paper) | ISBN 9780226437545 (pbk. : alk. paper) | ISBN 9780226437682 (e-book)
Subjects: LCSH: Orphans—Uganda—Social conditions. | Children of AIDS patients—Uganda—Social conditions. | Poor children—Uganda—social conditions. | Child welfare—Uganda. | AIDS (Disease)—Social aspects—Uganda.
Classification: LCC HV1347 .C44 2017 | DDC 305.23086/945—dc23
LC record available at https://lccn.loc.gov/2016029264

Dedicated to Dorothy Nang'wale Oulanyah (1970–2009)
and all grandmothers who care for children

In memory of my own grandmothers,
Eva Cheney (1923–2008) and Mabel Rocamora (1915–2014)

Contents

Abbreviations ix
Introduction 1

PART 1 Generations of HIV/AIDS, Orphanhood, and Intervention

1   A Generation of HIV/AIDS in Uganda   13
2   Orphanhood and the Conundrum of Humanitarian Intervention   24

PART 2 Beyond Checking the "Voice" Box: Children's Rights
and Participation in Development and Research

3   Children's Rights: Participation, Protectionism, and Citizenship   43
4   Getting Children's Perspectives: A Child- and Youth-Centered
    Participatory Approach   58

PART 3 Orphanhood in the Age of HIV and AIDS

5   Orphanhood, Poverty, and the Post-ARV Generation   87
6   Suffering, Silence, and Status: The Lived Experience of Orphanhood   107

PART 4 Blood Binds: The Transformation of
Kinship and the Politics of Adoption

7   Orphanhood and the Transformation of Kinship, Fosterage,
    and Children's Circulation Strategies   131
8   Orphanhood and the Politics of Adoption in Uganda   156

PART 5 Conclusion

9 HIV/AIDS Policy, "Orphan Addiction," and the Next Generation   181

Acknowledgments 189
Appendix: Children and Household Profiles by
Youth Research Assistant Focus Group, 2007–2009 191
Notes 215
References 221
Index 235

Abbreviations

ACRWC	African Charter on the Rights and Welfare of the Child
ART	antiretroviral therapy
ARV	antiretroviral
A-TRAIN	African Training, Research, and Innovation Network
CABA	children affected by AIDS
CAFO	Christian Alliance for Orphans
CBOs	community-based organizations
CHIFF	Children in Families First
CRC	Convention on the Rights of the Child
MDG	Millennium Development Goals
NGOs	nongovernmental organizations
OVC	orphans and vulnerable children
PEPFAR	President's Emergency Plan for AIDS Relief (US)
PMTCT	prevention of mother-to-child transmission
PTV	Protecting the Vulnerable (program of UNICEF)
RAs	research assistants
SAP	structural adjustment program
UCRNN	Uganda Child Rights NGO Network
UN	United Nations
UNAIDS	Joint United Nations Programme on HIV/AIDS
UNFPA	United Nations Population Fund, originally United Nations Fund for Population Activities
UNICEF	United Nations Children's Fund, originally United Nations International Children's Emergency Fund
USAID	United States Agency for International Development
UWESO	Uganda Women's Effort to Save Orphans
VCT	voluntary counseling and testing

Introduction

We are the young generation.
We are crying for our elders.
AIDS, AIDS has killed so many people . . .
Oh, no shouting, no advice:
Where shall we go?

SONG SUNG BY UGANDAN
GRADE SCHOOL CHILDREN

During the course of my research about childhood in Uganda since the 1990s, I have come across many children who have been orphaned. I often wondered how the loss of one or both parents would affect their life chances. Given the statistics coming out of aid and human development literature, their prospects were not good: when I started research for this book in 2007, the numbers of orphans in Uganda and other African nations were expected to double within the next five to seven years as the AIDS epidemic was reaching its apogee and killing off society's most productive (and reproductive) age group: their parents.[1]

Margaret was one of the many children I met who was living with extended family after her parents had both died.[2] She was the tallest girl in the fifth grade, with bright eyes and a gracious smile. She lived with her uncle because both her parents had already passed away. One Monday morning during a fieldwork visit to her school, she accosted me, saying she had been anxiously waiting all weekend to see me. She explained that her uncle had also passed away from AIDS complications the previous Friday. Her aunt was not her blood relative, and if Margaret stayed with her, her aunt said she could not guarantee that she could afford to pay Margaret's school fees. Three days after her uncle's death, Margaret, a twelve-year-old girl, was already soliciting alternative sources of support: might I be able to find someone to sponsor her, she asked?

Like many other children I would meet over the course of my research in Uganda, Margaret displayed exceptional resilience and agency in the fight for survival in the era of AIDS orphanhood. The children's song from which this book lends its title, however, conveys less resilience, and less hope. It is also ambiguous: it references the jeopardized social reproduction and threatened intergenerational relations of which the children who sing it are a part. But what is it really implying when it states that children are "crying for their elders"? Are they crying out of need, asking their elders to help them? Or are they crying out of sympathy for their elders, either their parents who have died or the grandparents who are taking on the responsibility of caring for orphans? I got different answers from those I asked—from the teachers who taught it to classrooms of children to the children who learned and hummed it—each giving an interpretation based on their own experiences with AIDS.

The rest of the refrain suggests that it is likely the former, but because "AIDS has killed so many people," some children cry for the loss of their elders who would otherwise be there to shout (raise concern) and guide them in life. The last line implies confusion over where to go to find solace or support. I wondered whether orphaned children really felt they no longer had anyone to turn to—or maybe the last line, "Where shall we go?" is a more general expression of worry over their own futures. This research was an opportunity to unravel the riddle.

Encounters with children like Margaret and hearing songs like these led me to my current research questions: How do children actually experience HIV/AIDS and orphanhood? How has AIDS influenced the social fabric of children's lives, especially in terms of intergenerational relationships? How has humanitarian intervention on behalf of children orphaned by AIDS affected the broader social circumstances in which children grow up? What survival strategies do families, communities, and children themselves employ to ameliorate the circumstances of orphanhood, particularly in the age of HIV and AIDS?

After many years of longitudinal ethnographic study on HIV/AIDS and orphanhood, I have to start here with an apology and a disclaimer about misleading the reader: in investigating orphanhood, I was repeatedly drawn back to the conclusion that it is not really AIDS or orphanhood per se that posed the greatest adversity to children but in fact structural challenges such as poverty and lack of quality education that exacerbate the circumstances of orphanhood—and from which a focus on orphanhood itself can actually divert attention (Henderson 2006; Meintjes and Giese 2006). I considered shifting the focus of the book away from orphanhood to child poverty more generally, but I realized that if I had labeled the book as being about anything other than orphanhood, I risked turning the discussion away from the misappropriation of such terms as *orphans* and *orphanhood*, as well as merely preaching to the converted, such that the book would fail to speak to the international audience that continues to place a reifying emphasis on orphans and orphanhood in isolation rather than on broader structures of childhood adversity. So I chose to keep orphanhood as my primary analytic object, if only to inhabit the contradictions that it presents to children's lives and unpack these contradictions for the reader.

My main argument in this book is that orphans and vulnerable children are constructed categories, created and propagated by the development and humanitarian industrial complex, that do not ultimately hold together within the social contexts of children's lives. This because they address just one of many aspects of children's lived experiences and identities and do not always encompass the single—or even most important—aspect of their vulnerability. As children and their caregivers tell it, it is not orphanhood itself but its intersections with other personal, social, and political circumstances and structural factors that adversely affect children's life chances. Indeed, a number of scholars have written that the AIDS pandemic has been similarly misconstrued (Stillwaggon 2006; Fassin 2007b), but I wish to make a related point that a focus on AIDS has also obscured the many other causes of orphanhood. And while others have argued that orphanhood as a created category for intervention—though often well-meaning—ultimately misdirects those interventions toward a singular 'label' and away from children and their families' broader social and material realities (Foster, Levine, and Williamson 2005; Henderson 2006; Meintjes and Giese 2006), this book describes in ethnographic detail the longitudinal consequences of such prioritization, considering the social, cultural, and political implications for Ugandan children and their families.

Conceptual and Methodological Considerations in the Study of AIDS Orphanhood

CRITICAL CHILDREN'S STUDIES

My departure point for this text is critical children's studies. Leena Alanen has observed—and I concur—that children's studies, having grown into its own as a field of inquiry, has reached a point at which a "normative turn" is needed to make a positive difference in children's lives (Alanen 2011). There is a growing dissatisfaction in children's studies—at least among those who entered the field for the betterment of children's lives—that we are not making the policy or even the academic impact that we would like. Part of this dissatisfaction has to do with a persistent ghettoization of children's studies: much as women's studies, despite its growth as a field of inquiry in the 1970s and 1980s, continued to suffer marginalization in the patriarchal academy, children's studies also continues to remain a "side subject" to what is considered "serious" academic inquiry. We certainly can be accused of a considerable degree of self-segregation and even navel-gazing, but I also have seen that the failure to find audience with other disciplines has to do with their reluctance to take children's studies seriously. The fact that we continue to emulate the very existence of children's agency, for example, indicates that although we are thoroughly convinced that children are people in their own right, we still feel the need to convince others of this truism before we can move on to discuss more substantive issues such as what constrains that agency and how children negotiate those obstacles.

Women's studies encountered similar challenges, but we in childhood studies seem to be having a harder time of it, perhaps because we have the dual disadvantage of having to overcome prejudices about both gender and age. By this I mean that childhood studies is seen in the academy not only as an infantilized subject by virtue of its young objects of inquiry but as a women's concern (in a still-very-patriarchal academy) by virtue of the fact that the field is dominated by female scholars. Worse, the assumption is all too often that women's intellectual interest in children is somehow linked to their own biological imperatives as mothers—or in the case of female scholars who do not have children, that it serves as a proxy for not having fulfilled that biological imperative. This assumption, of course, is ludicrous, but it is not uncommon for female scholars of childhood to be questioned about the connections between their research and their personal reproductive decisions, which in itself is telling of the patriarchal state of the academy, and it is one area where children's studies needs to continue to challenge the status quo. As archaeologist Jane Baxter succinctly put it, "Feminized research topics are often . . . seen as 'less than' other topics, perspectives, and ideas in a discipline. The quiet assumption children are only a viable/interesting topic in archaeology because it is of interest to women working out their interests/issues in motherhood diminishes children as scholarly subjects and women as scholars" (Baxter 2015). This diminishment is also evidenced in the persistent rejection of child-related topics from journals and meetings focusing on nonchildhood disciplines. It is all the more vexing when one sees conference presentations and articles from scholars who identify with other disciplines—but whose work solidly deals with child and youth issues—fail to acknowledge and even roundly ignore sound scholarship from children and youth studies that would inform their work. Though childhood studies scholars seem eager and able to borrow from other disciplines to inform their work, it has not become a two-way street. My generation could not study squarely within children's studies, but now that departments are being established, it will be interesting to see whether children's studies becomes more or less integrated in the academy.

The same could be said of childhood studies' relationship with policy makers. Policy is another male-dominated field, where "evidence-based" is often interpreted in positivist terms of numbers and "hard" sciences—also seen as masculine compared to the "soft" social sciences such as childhood studies that focus more on social practice and processes of meaning making. The nuance such social research inquiry produces is usually seen as a distraction by policy makers who want black-and-white figures that can show them the "progress" and "effectiveness" of policy decisions. A good example is human development research, whose central narrative, developed primarily by economists, has sold the idea that children are important only in terms of return on investment—that is, as human capital. Further, as I have argued before (Cheney 2007b), this approach fails to recognize the current contributions of the young to national development—and having children's citizenship relegated to the future frustrates young people to no end. Jo Boyden of the Young Lives Project[3]—one of the biggest longitudinal, international studies of childhood poverty to date, led by the University of Oxford's Department of International Development—has argued that this ideology has also served to further a global neoliberal agenda facilitating the retreat of the state from its responsibilities toward citizens, including children. Nonetheless, this powerful human development discourse captivates policy makers—despite evidence from Young Lives that challenges human development assumptions such as those that developmental delays in early childhood are irreversible, that Western-style formal education is a panacea for poverty, or that girls are universally more disadvantaged than boys (Boyden 2015). The human development discourse captivates policy makers not only because the human capital approach offers a simplistic narrative with apparently clear solutions to child poverty but also because social research, while it justly critiques this narrative, too often stops short of offering effective alternatives.

Boyden suggests that childhood studies needs to overcome the micro/macro conundrum by paying more attention to, for example, political economy approaches to childhood. But despite having personally conducted political economic analyses of childhood for years (Cheney 2007b, 2014b; Cheney and Rotabi 2014), it does not seem to have taken hold—precisely, perhaps, because it introduces nuances that challenge the dominant ideologies of human development theory. Again, however, I am not convinced that it is a matter of scholars of childhood studies failing to reach out to policy makers so much as a failure of policy makers to embrace and take seriously childhood studies.

Can childhood studies ever be taken more seriously? If we want to go beyond the box-ticking of children's rights, voice, acknowledging agency, and justifying the importance of our own work, we need a more critical and reflexive childhood studies that problematizes the norms, approaches, and practices—not just in the phenomena we observe but in our own research and indeed our own institutions and the academy at large. It is also for this reason—the need to address power, patriarchy, and participation—that I have chosen in this study to employ a youth participatory research model, upon which I elaborate in part 2.

POSTHUMANITARIANISM

To establish the necessary critical social justice stance on children's studies, I also wish to bring it into conversation with postdevelopment and posthumanitarianism literature, in which a depoliticized sense of solidarity with suffering others converges with the marketization of humanitarianism to instrumentalize it as a project of self-cultivation (Chouliaraki 2013). My aim here is to problematize the figure of the "orphan." Orphans are arguably the quintessential poster children of humanitarian aid campaigns. Late humanitarian consciousness is in many ways founded on the image of the suffering child, an image meant to urge potential private donors toward action (Chouliaraki 2013). However, as Liisa Malkki has noted, children often symbolically act in humanitarian appeals as "generic human moral subjects . . . not as culturally or socially specific *persons*" (Malkki 2010, 66). This representation is what facilitates a sense of moral solidarity between donors and recipients, but one that is premised on inequality. By questioning the reasons for the persistence of child rescue narratives that underpin charitable and humanitarian interventions—not only on behalf of children themselves but on behalf of children who act as proxies for entire vulnerable populations and ambassadors of the future—I aim to highlight the adverse consequences, some of which can actually extend and create new categories of child vulnerability rather than ameliorate it. This persistence of child rescue narratives goes back to the conflation of poverty with orphanhood, and as Didier Fassin has described it, "the fallacious presentation of children as parentless, their depiction as victims" (Fassin 2013, 125) cannot be separated from the phenomenon of African AIDS orphanhood. Otherwise, this reifying move allows us to separate children from the broader social networks in which they are embedded—and vice versa—creating a depoliticized and infantilized notion of "the deserving poor" through the figure of the orphan. As Feldman and Ticktin point out, "When only the absolutely innocent elicit care, giving, and empathy . . . our solidarity and ability to create lasting peace remains dependent on a mirage and [is] thus easily thwarted" (2010, 15). But scholars can fall into the same pitfalls they identify if they too fail to consider how those who are made objects of humanitarian intervention respond and adapt to such prevalent and powerful discourses. Childhood studies could thus play a valuable role in informing posthumanitarianism studies about the ways these discourses actually play out in children's lives, not least because of the ways in which children incorporate or resist such discourses. I therefore use ethnography to demonstrate that orphans are individuals within families and communities, who also respond strategically to dominant depictions of orphans, sometimes resisting and sometimes interpellating the categorization of "orphan," even as an ironically empowering identity. Grounding these discourses in the actual lives of children thus opens the possibility of "going beyond the spectacle in order to recuperate a positive view of the theatre [of dramaturgical consciousness] as moral education" (Chouliaraki 2013, 43).

GENERATIONS

Aside from drawing on critical childhood studies, a generational analysis helps place the stories of orphanhood told in this book in relational context. Because generation is an essentially relational category, it resists the reification of children and orphanhood. A generational analysis also helps place Ugandan orphanhood in its specific sociohistorical moment, which in this case is part of the trajectory of HIV/AIDS and its treatment following the apogee of the AIDS epidemic in Uganda. Specifically, I argue that the youth the age of those who participated in this project as research assistants and the children the age of those with whom they did ethnographic fieldwork comprise what I am calling here the "post-ARV [antiretroviral] generation." By reinvoking Karl Mannheim's notion of generation as a social category punctuated by national and even global events that mark their common experience of childhood and solidify their identity as a generation (Mannheim 1982), I highlight how the young can be the ones to "rewrite the rules" in the given historical moment by choosing how they respond to these defining events (Woodman and Wyn 2014, 8). After painting the larger picture of the era in which these children have grown, I ethnographically detail how children and youth try to make a way forward by negotiating various social constraints and opportunities. This approach may help get past the stalemate of agency debates in childhood studies, where we are still trying to convince policy makers that children are people—since it is not a question of whether or not children and youth have agency but how they wield it under particular circumstances.

How the Book Is Structured

The first part, "Generations of HIV/AIDS, Orphanhood, and Intervention," provides the macro context against which African AIDS orphanhood has been constructed by placing HIV/AIDS and orphanhood in the broad socio-historical backdrop against which the children and their interlocutors in this book have lived their lives. I argue that delayed recognition of the impending "orphan crisis" that UNICEF (the United Nations Children's Fund, originally the United Nations International Children's Emergency Fund) and others believed would soon follow the apogee of the AIDS epidemic in Africa, while it never fully came to pass, irrevocably changed the field of humanitarian intervention and child protection in Uganda and many other parts of sub-Saharan Africa. This humanitarian influence has shaped the context in which the children described in this book have grown up—either by inclusion or by exclusion. It also forms the rationale for this research. Chapter 1, "A Generation of HIV/AIDS in Uganda," shows how the trajectory of the HIV/AIDS epidemic—particularly the rollout of antiretroviral treatment—maps onto the lives of the young people in this generation. Chapter 2, "Orphanhood and the Conundrum of Humanitarian Intervention," draws on critical humanitarian studies and a political economic approach to orphanhood to reconsider the dynamics of childhood vulnerability in the Ugandan context, from policy to practice.

Part 2, "Beyond Checking the 'Voice' Box: Children's Rights and Participation in Development and Research," discusses the theoretical and methodological approaches employed in gathering the data for this book, specifically a meaningful approach to children's rights and youth participatory research. I discuss the issues that arise in the process of doing child- and youth-centered research, highlighting the importance of longitudinal ethnographic fieldwork that allows for the emergence of children's points of view without reifying children's "voices." To avoid paying lip service to giving "voice" to children, their rights, or their empowerment, this volume calls for a participatory approach that involves young people from design to data collection to analysis. I detail the research design I used that drew on the work of youth research assistants (RAs)—the youths who participated in my earlier study—as an example of how participatory research with young people, while not without its challenges, can yield more authentic information about the lives of children. Part 2 includes chapter 3, "Children's Rights: Participation, Protectionism, and Citizenship," and chapter 4, "Getting Children's Perspectives: A Child- and Youth-Centered Participatory Approach."

Part 3, "Orphanhood in the Age of HIV and AIDS," chronicles some of the experiences of the children in the study community (see the appendix for complete profiles of each child in the youth RA focus groups) and highlights the conclusions drawn from the ethnographic data collected by the youth research assistants. It starts, however, with the youth research assistants' own experiences of growing up in this era of HIV/AIDS in chapter 5, "Orphanhood, Poverty, and the Post-ARV Generation." By continuing their life histories, which were featured in my book *Pillars of the Nation* (Cheney 2007b), I highlight how AIDS orphanhood in the post-ARV generation is still compounded by other structural vulnerabilities. Through updating their stories, we get to know not only how orphanhood has affected these young people over time but also how they have responded to the challenges posed by it.

In the second chapter of part 3—chapter 6, "Suffering, Silence, and Status: The Lived Experience of Orphanhood"—I discuss the seemingly contradictory stigma surrounding AIDS orphanhood in families and local communities. The chapter deals with orphanhood as lived experience, highlighting the role of HIV/AIDS as a primary cause of orphan suffering, which compounds problems of poverty and insecurity. Despite Uganda's leadership in the 1980s and 1990s in addressing HIV, stigma and silences around HIV as the cause of orphanhood are still profound, and they adversely affect children's abilities to express their grief at the losses of life around them. At the same time as silences around AIDS are meant to protect children, they can prove problematic for the future trajectories of orphans, who are at higher risk of HIV infection, or—for those who are already HIV-positive—are at risk of spreading HIV when their own HIV status is concealed from them. As these silences and stilted expressions of suffering are also problematic for research, I include in this chapter a discussion of ethical and methodological challenges for the study of childhood suffering in the context of AIDS orphanhood.

Part 4, "Blood Binds: The Transformation of Kinship and the Politics of Adoption," traces several important social transformations in the Ugandan institutions of family and community that have affected children as a result of AIDS orphanhood and persistent poverty. These social transformations have posed new challenges, but so has the evolution of humanitarianism on behalf of children—particularly through the emergence of an "orphan movement" abroad that, while well meaning, has actually exacerbated the "orphan crisis" it wishes to ameliorate. In this section, *blood* acts as a central theme, both as a metaphor of relatedness and as a substance that binds orphaned children in social relationships with kin that have created some more conundrums for the provision of orphan care. First, in chapter 7, "Orphanhood and the Transformation of Kinship, Fosterage, and Children's Circulation Strategies," I argue that the AIDS pandemic has set in motion some significant transformations in the formation of kinship, not only in terms of who cares for whom but in terms of obligation and affect among kin.

One might ask whether adoption is a feasible response to mass orphan-hood, and while all available research shows that it is neither an efficient nor a typically appropriate response, chapter 8, "Orphanhood and the Politics of Adoption in Uganda," chronicles the recent ascent of a charitable "orphan in-dustrial complex" in Uganda. This problematic yet powerful movement is not only confronting Ugandans' conceptions of "blood" obligations but is also undermining child protection by creating avenues for the unnecessary insti-tutionalization of children. The proliferation of orphanages is thus making "orphans" of tens of thousands of children with families for the purposes of charitable intervention and has opened up the country to child trafficking for purposes of intercountry adoption.

Finally, the part 5 conclusion in its chapter 9, "HIV/AIDS Policy, Orphan Addiction, and the Next Generation," details the state of HIV/AIDS and or-phanhood today, evaluating young Ugandans' prospects for the future. The news is not very good, especially given the resurgence of HIV prevalence, limited resources for delivering services to orphans, and the ways in which those resources and services are being used to further certain political and ideological agendas. But young people of the post-ARV generation see trans-formation in their time and still hold out hope for the next generation. I end with suggestions for approaches to further policy reform and call for more child and youth participatory research.

PART ONE

Generations of HIV/AIDS, Orphanhood, and Intervention

A Generation of HIV/AIDS in Uganda

In her edited volume *Second Chances: Surviving AIDS in Uganda*, Susan R. Whyte and her colleagues describe the outcomes of a longitudinal study on the progression of the AIDS epidemic in Uganda through the concept of a "biogeneration," a cohort of people whose life experiences are "defined by the management of an epidemic and an innovative package of care" (Whyte 2014, 2). Whyte goes on to describe the history of public health interventions that accompanied the spread of HIV/AIDS and eventually turned the tide of the disease—not only through prevention but through the introduction of treatment, particularly antiretroviral therapy (ART). ART transformed the diagnosis of HIV from an automatic death sentence to a manageable disease. As Whyte notes, Uganda is a good country in which to follow AIDS's first generation of survivors (2014, 4) because Uganda was one of the countries first and hardest hit by the epidemic. The Ugandan government was also the first to respond in a concerted, multisectoral way. Whyte observes that "the first generation to benefit from ART in Uganda had been more exposed than citizens of other eastern and southern African states to massive information campaigns and a multitude of AIDS projects well before effective treatment rolled out" (2014, 4).

These campaigns helped bring about declines in both the prevalence and the incidence of HIV infections. The advent of ART has thus also punctuated the lives of the children with whom I have worked since 2000. HIV testing became available in Uganda in 1990, the time around which the children whose life histories I chronicled in *Pillars of the Nation* (Cheney 2007b) and who served as youth research assistants for this project were born. The prevention of mother-to-child transmission (PMTCT) of HIV treatment became widely available in 2000, the year in which I began fieldwork for *Pillars*. ART

The Post-ARV Generation

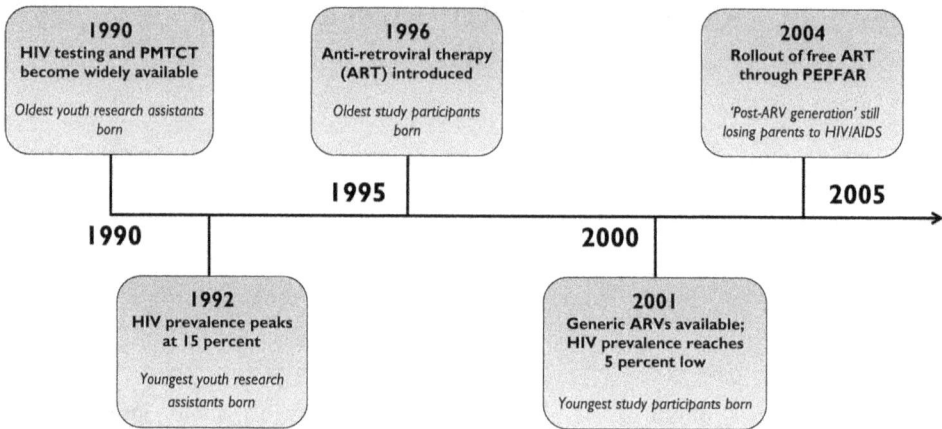

1990	1996	2004
HIV testing and PMTCT become widely available	**Anti-retroviral therapy (ART) introduced**	**Rollout of free ART through PEPFAR**
Oldest youth research assistants born	*Oldest study participants born*	*'Post-ARV generation' still losing parents to HIV/AIDS*

1990   **1995**   **2000**   **2005**

1992	2001
HIV prevalence peaks at 15 percent	**Generic ARVs available; HIV prevalence reaches 5 percent low**
Youngest youth research assistants born	*Youngest study participants born*

FIGURE 1. Time line of the post-ARV generation.

was introduced in Uganda in 1996, but it was far too expensive for everyone but the very wealthy. When generics came on the market in 2001, however, the possibility of long-term survival through the medical management of HIV became available to a greater number of Ugandans. And when the US President's Emergency Plan for AIDS Relief (PEPFAR) made Uganda one of its top three aid recipients in 2004, many thousands more started receiving free ART (Whyte 2014, 5–7). The availability of treatment affected the cohort of children with whom we did youth participatory research for this volume, who were born between 1996 and 2002 (see time line in fig. 1). We might well call this generation the "*post-ARV generation*," then.

The biogeneration on which Whyte and her colleagues focused were people around thirty to forty years old at the time of research in the early part of the first decade of the twenty-first century. While "the notion of generation invites us to inquire into the distinctive consciousness that characterizes those who experience fateful historical events" (Whyte 2014, 13), the consciousness of children is often overlooked or discounted. Whyte and her associates opted to concentrate on those who had reached adulthood by the time treatment—what they identify as the defining moment of the era—was made widely available in the first few years of the twenty-first century. Yet HIV/AIDS may actually have had the greatest impact on the children who were born and came of age in the wake of the development of such treatments. While the young children we talked to during intensive fieldwork from 2007 to 2009 may not have had a "generational consciousness" related to the spread and treatment of AIDS at the time (most were five to ten years old), it has clearly had an impact on their lives, especially those for whose parents' ARV treatment became accessible too late to prolong their lives. This book is thus dedicated to understanding how children of the post-ARV generation, particularly orphaned children, were affected by and experienced the same post-ART era of the HIV/AIDS pandemic described by Whyte et al. I start first with an overview of the broader national and international developments in HIV/AIDS treatment—as they relate to orphans—to set the stage for the latter parts of the book, which deal with the more local and household-level social contexts of orphans' lives.

The Course of the HIV/AIDS Epidemic in Uganda

Numerous sources have detailed how Uganda, being at the epicenter of the African AIDS pandemic, showed relatively early government leadership in seeking international assistance to identify and combat the disease (Thornton 2008; Seeley 2014). Government's attention was initially on prevention, as no cure or treatment was known; it launched major public education campaigns and managed to help Uganda become one of two countries (the other being Senegal, whose AIDS epidemic never reached the same proportions) to reverse its HIV prevalence rate from a peak of about 15 percent (and 30 percent among pregnant women tested in prenatal clinics) in 1992 to a low of about 5 percent in 2001. Some countries still have not embraced leadership in AIDS prevention, and that decision has had far more disastrous consequences for them.

Scholars have variously theorized the reasons for Uganda's apparent success versus the failures of other nations to tackle the rise in HIV/AIDS infections in the 1980s and 1990s. In her book *The Invisible Cure: Why We Are Losing the Fight against AIDS in Africa* (2007), Helen Epstein posits that Ugandans' early success in battling AIDS was due to their acceptance of the vector of transmission and subsequent behavior change amid concurrent sexual relationships—overlapping long-term relationships—that typically occur in African communities. Robert Thornton's sexual network theory similarly posits that AIDS circulated in comparatively tight sexual networks in Uganda, where understandings of AIDS were indigenized early in the epidemic (Thornton 2008). Unlike Epstein, however, Thornton believes that rather than attributing the reduction in AIDS infections solely to individual behavior change, much more cultural and social shifts in sexual networks are also responsible. Janet Seeley's historical overview, *HIV and East Africa:*

Thirty Years in the Shadow of an Epidemic, argues that "sexual activity occurs in the context of a person's life course. But this broader context is often overlooked in the urge to identify individuals in particular 'risk groups'" (2014, 4). Seeley therefore sets to the task of contextualizing the spread of HIV and AIDS in relation to social, historical, and economic events in the region's recent history, noting variations and fluctuations across time and space.

One aspect that is generally agreed on is that Uganda was unique in its early recognition of—and intervention in—AIDS as an urgent matter of public health. This quick response accordingly yielded early successes, especially with PMTCT drastically reducing the national rate of transmission to children during pregnancy. Less discussed, however, is the adverse effect this treatment has had on children who survive and are orphaned as their mothers and fathers succumb to AIDS. As the orphan population in Africa exploded in the 1990s, extended families that are traditionally responsible for orphan care were trying to meet the needs of their families as people died before raising their children. International and government interventions thus centered on strengthening existing social safety nets and bolstering their resilience. Uganda tackled the disease itself first, but the response to the fact of children becoming orphaned came later. *AIDS, in other words, was treated first and foremost as a medical phenomenon, to the detriment of attention toward its devastating social effects, such as mass orphanhood.*

In the late 1990s and the early twenty-first century, UNICEF (the United Nations Children's Fund, originally the United Nations International Children's Emergency Fund) increased efforts to highlight the plight of children affected by AIDS by adopting a purposefully broad definition of an orphan as any "child under 18 years of age whose mother, father, or both parents have died" (UNICEF 2006, 4). By this definition, UNICEF could claim that an estimated 53 million sub-Saharan African children had been orphaned by 2006—30 percent (15.7 million) of them by AIDS (UNICEF 2006, iv). In turn, many international nongovernmental organizations (NGOs) and charities have focused on the plight of AIDS orphans—then children affected by AIDS (CABA), orphans and vulnerable children (OVC), and so on (see chapter 2 for a brief etymology of orphan terminology). But this humanitarianism often comes with adverse consequences, intended or unintended.

The way UNICEF's definition inflated orphan numbers led to an outcry about an imminent "orphan crisis" that threatened to overwhelm extended-family systems and leave thousands of children without care. Following UNICEF, scholars and practitioners began to use the term *orphan crisis* both widely and uncritically (Guest 2003; Roby and Shaw 2006; Drah 2012). Yet UNICEF's broad definition can distort local definitions by singling out orphaned children as particularly vulnerable despite widespread extended-family social safety nets (Meintjes and Giese 2006; Sherr et al. 2008). Nonetheless, international responses in the 1980s and 1990s tended to focus on the "orphan" in isolation from the extended family, and even from the broader community. While this portrayal elicits a variety of charitable, humanitarian responses out of sympathy for parentless children, inflating orphan numbers to attract scarce resources ultimately does little to remedy the structural issues that lead to orphanhood in the first place (Cheney 2010). I return to this point in chapter 2.

The trajectory of the African AIDS pandemic is still playing out as the number of orphans requiring care continues to increase. There are several reasons for this. First, there is a lag between peak HIV prevalence (the proportion of cases relative to the total population) and death due to AIDS, which means the number of orphans increases even after HIV prevalence drops—but HIV prevalence in fact rose again in Uganda from 6.4 percent in 2005 to 7.3 percent in 2011, and the incidence, or probability of occurrence, also rose slightly until 2012, when it began to decline again (Uganda AIDS Commission 2014, vii). Though Uganda has seen a dramatic drop in the number of children newly infected with HIV as a result of PMTCT rollout, new infection rates remain high among the adult population (Uganda AIDS Commission 2014), which means that the probability that Ugandan children will continue to be orphaned by AIDS also remains high.

Second, the coverage of antiretroviral therapy has still not been sufficient to prevent the deaths of all parents. According to the World Bank, only 38 percent of all Ugandans who needed ART were in fact receiving it in 2013.[1]

Third, the ART coverage for children is even lower: in 2011, only 21 percent of the HIV-positive Ugandan children ranging in age from infancy through age fourteen were receiving ART in 2011 (UNICEF 2012). Though coverage remains insufficient,[2] more HIV-positive children receiving ART also means that those children, who would otherwise likely have died by age five (Sikstrom 2014, 47), are now living to adulthood—but often as orphans. Such survival occurs because most were infected perinatally, so their parents may since have died while the children have survived (a situation true of all four HIV-positive children in the present study). Even as adult mortality drastically fell following the rollout of ART, HIV-positive children's survival inflates orphan numbers.

In other words, only recently have efforts turned attention toward orphans as an unfortunate outcome of the epidemic, and only recently have ARVs been made more widely available to people with HIV, which has helped prolong their lives long enough for them to raise their children. But ARVs have come too late to stem the proliferation of orphans in the early twenty-first century. In the meantime, extended families and communities who were caring for nonbiological children were disproportionately strained, leading to increased overall poverty.

Community-based organizations (CBOs) and NGOs were the first organized responders to the proliferation of AIDS orphans. Many CBOs started with small interventions for the children they saw suffering in their own communities, particularly when they saw that children were heading households themselves or taking to the streets due to lack of parental care. Despite small-scale community efforts to attend to orphan needs, however, orphans and vulnerable children remained largely invisible in early HIV/AIDS care, prevention, and treatment programs. Government response to the orphan crisis was delayed, perhaps relying on extended family networks to continue absorbing orphans until it became clear that these traditional means of orphan support were being stretched beyond their capacity by the AIDS pandemic.

Despite pressure from below, the development of national OVC policies was largely the result of consultation with international donors and NGOs. The Rapid Assessment, Analysis, and Action Planning (RAAAP) initiative —established by the United States Agency for International Development (USAID), UNICEF, the Joint United Nations Programme on HIV/AIDS (UNAIDS), and the World Food Programme—coordinated the efforts of seventeen sub-Saharan African countries' strategic planning to meet the needs of the growing numbers of orphans in their countries in 2003 (POLICY Project 2005). Although these countries developed national plans of action, only six African countries had developed national policies for orphan care by the end of 2003 (Roby and Shaw 2006, 201). Uganda did not implement its policy until 2004—twelve years after peak HIV prevalence. Though national OVC policies thus happened to some extent by default, their establishment still holds promise for the 17.7 million children worldwide who have been orphaned by AIDS—10.5 million of them in Eastern and Southern Africa, and 1.1 million in Uganda alone (UNAIDS 2013; UNICEF 2014)—that their governments and civil society are taking leadership on the issue, as any policy that focuses on child well-being is better late than never.

Enter PEPFAR

Uganda's rollout of its OVC policy was also the year that US President George W. Bush's administration rolled out the President's Emergency Plan for AIDS Relief (PEPFAR). PEPFAR was established in 2004 with a $15 billion budget to treat and prevent HIV and AIDS in Africa. Uganda was one of the target countries and one of the top three recipients of funding (Whyte 2014, 7). Despite the incredible investment PEPFAR made in public health in Africa, however, it was not without its politics.

At an African Studies Association meeting I attended during the course of this study, I met one of the scholars who had been hired by the US government to research and compile a report on which it would base the initial PEPFAR budget allocation.[3] He told me how his team was first sent to Uganda for several months of fact-finding about the effective measures Ugandans had taken to reduce their HIV infection rate—after which they would move on to conduct similar research in six other sub-Saharan African countries. The team went north, south, east, and west in the country talking to patients, doctors, policy makers, and others, gathering data on Uganda's HIV "success story." After the initial gathering of data, some PEPFAR representatives from Washington, DC, flew in to Kampala to receive a progress report from the research team. As the team ran through its presentation in a conference room at the Sheraton Hotel, they listed some of the treatment and prevention methods that had been shown to be most successful in Uganda, including the prevention of mother-to-child transmission, the creation of AIDS support groups, voluntary counseling and testing (VCT), condom use—"Stop!" interrupted a PEPFAR representative with a raised, open palm. "You're *not* going to talk about condoms." The team was shocked and baffled by this interruption; the team members rebutted that they had gathered definitive evidence that condoms, when used correctly, were a substantial factor in the reduction of HIV prevalence in Uganda. But the Washington representatives insisted that they were not going to entertain any suggestions about condom use when it came to prevention. They were adamant that PEPFAR prevention programs would emphasize abstinence approaches, evidence or no evidence. Some team members tried to negotiate while others broke down in tears of frustration that scientific inquiry was apparently once again being hijacked for political purposes.

The research team continued to plead, but the representatives finally said that if the research team insisted on talking about condom use, they would cancel the rest of the seven-country fact-finding mission. The team insisted on the integrity of the members' own reputations as researchers, so the rest of the research mission was canceled. Some researchers threw their hands up, walked out, and went straight to the airport while others sat stunned for a time. The team member told me that the representatives returned to Washington, DC, and commissioned a member of the Presidential Advisory Council on HIV/AIDS to write the report without taking any of their research into account.

PEPFAR has been touted in popular media as an altruistic and over-whelming success (in 2008, the US Congress reauthorized the program to the tune of $48 billion), but many observers have since written critiques of PEPFAR's latent politics (Susser 2009; Thornton 2008). While PEPFAR has received accolades for extending the lives of millions of people on PEPFAR-funded ARV treatments (including several children in this study), it has done so by supporting a mosaic of projects, from secular and faith-based NGOs to state and regional efforts. Whyte points out that not only was these programs' sustainability dependent on the continuance of foreign funding but that "PEPFAR . . . did not exclusively or even primarily target the public health system. In some ways, the NGO and international donor AIDS projects un-dermined the government health care system by drawing health workers away to better-paid jobs" (Whyte 2014, 7). Further, PEPFAR's privileging of faith-based organizations also imposed a conservative, religious approach to prevention that continues to promote unsustainable, moralizing abstinence-only programs for youth while discouraging such proven strategies as con-dom use (Human Rights Watch/Africa 2005). One-third of the original al-location of prevention money under PEPFAR was earmarked by Congress for abstinence and fidelity programming—despite its previously proven failures in US sex education (di Mauro and Joffe 2008; Kendall 2013). Despite the US government's reauthorizations of PEPFAR and the Global Fund to Fight AIDS, Tuberculosis, and Malaria that help maintain ART, the budget for ab-stinence and fidelity programming was only cut in 2015 from $47 million to $21 million (McNeil 2015).

The distribution of lifesaving and prolonging ART notwithstanding, the PEPFAR approach to prevention has threatened the lives of the next genera-tion. According to PEPFAR Watch, a rights monitoring group, no PEPFAR funding recipient can distribute condoms to people younger than fifteen years old, keeping "life saving tools from younger at-risk youth."[4] Human Rights Watch published a 2005 report on PEPFAR-funded abstinence-only programs in Uganda, claiming that their implementation has violated chil-dren's rights by denying them access to accurate information about HIV infection. The report asserts, among other things, that the program spreads misinformation about prevention measures: "Draft secondary-school materi-als state falsely that latex condoms have microscopic pores that can be per-meated by HIV, and that pre-marital sex is a form of 'deviance.' HIV/AIDS rallies sponsored by the U.S. government spread similar falsehoods."[5] The re-port also details how faith-based proabstinence institutions suddenly gained access to incredible amounts of funding they could use, despite having no experience in AIDS education or counseling, to further their proselytizing under the guise of public health. In fact, the Bush administration had laid the groundwork in 2002 by establishing a Center for Faith-Based and Community Initiatives within the USAID, "the purpose of which was to remove any obstacles to community and faith-based organizations' participation in USAID programs and promote their involvement 'to the greatest extent possible'" (Human Rights Watch/Africa 2005, 44). While not all funding went to faith-based organizations, initial qualification for PEPFAR funding was also made contingent on recipients' pledge that they opposed prostitution (Susser 2009, 64)—which effectively excluded sex workers, some of the most marginalized yet highly affected groups of people, from the benefits of PEPFAR programming. Nevertheless, PEPFAR's reach has been influential and has thus played a large role in shaping the young people of this generation's attitudes and perceptions of HIV and AIDS.

A Fragmented Response to Orphanhood

Global efforts to stem the AIDS epidemic coincided with neoliberal reforms in the aid industry, decentralization in nations such as Uganda, and the rise of NGOs in the 1990s (Bernal and Grewal 2014). The convergence of these events further threatened to fragment efforts to conquer HIV and AIDS orphanhood. Many African countries' action plans acknowledged that there was a high rate of duplication of OVC services and little communication or collaboration between service delivery organizations at the various levels. A 2009 survey by the NGO Viva revealed that there were more than five hundred organizations in Kampala alone working on orphan issues,[6] and yet little was being accomplished on a broad scale. The Ugandan government has therefore stepped back in by creating an OVC Secretariat under the Ministry of Gender, Labour, and Social Development to oversee the organizations already working on OVC issues. Under the mandate of the 2008 National OVC Policy, the OVC Secretariat liaised with UNICEF, the Uganda AIDS Commission, and others to rein in community-based and nongovernmental organizations under their umbrella to streamline services. But with the pervasiveness of NGOs, the response is still largely uncoordinated.

Although the creation of orphan policy was a positive sign based on the lessons learned at the grassroots level, the problem of implementation within the current structure remains vexing. My sense was that the people I talked with during my fieldwork—from UNICEF to the OVC Secretariat to NGO staff to grandmothers caring for orphans—are genuinely concerned for children's welfare, despite their limited resources for delivering services to orphans. On the other hand, the ways in which those resources tend to get siphoned off by the very people who are supposed to be looking out for orphans is equally disturbing and its effect on children understudied. Douglas Webb has suggested that "following a cohort of orphans over a short period could provide data that will draw attention to this highly vulnerable yet relatively invisible population" (2005, 236). Taking up Webb's suggestion, this book therefore focuses on the implications of both the AIDS pandemic and OVC policy for orphan well-being, particularly from the perspectives of children and caregivers.

An AIDS-Free Generation?

This book is about a generation of children—specifically children who have lost their parents to AIDS—who have never known a world without AIDS and thus experience both its burdens and its normalization. At the same time, if we take a Mannheimian approach to generational analysis to frame these children as a cohort bound together by a defining event, that event would be the rollout of ART from roughly 2004 to 2007 (fieldwork for this volume was conducted from 2007 to 2009, with follow-up visits from 2011 to 2015), making them the post-ARV generation.

Following a statement in 2011 by US secretary of state Hillary Rodham Clinton that the world was at the point for the first time in history where an AIDS-free generation was in sight, at the 2012 International AIDS Conference, Secretary Clinton called on PEPFAR under the Obama administration to outline how the United States would contribute to achieving this goal. According to a November 2012 US State Department press release coinciding with the release of the *PEPFAR Blueprint: Creating an AIDS-Free Generation*, "Secretary Clinton defined an AIDS-free generation as one where virtually no children are born with HIV; where, as these children become teenagers and adults, they are at far lower risk of becoming infected than they would be today; and where those who do acquire HIV have access to treatment that helps prevent them from developing AIDS and passing the virus on to others."[7]

PEPFAR and other international NGOs are still struggling to meet these goals. But as this generation of children infected with HIV begins to survive and live longer, HIV-positive children become both emblematic of the success of the fight against AIDS and a threat to it in that they may survive to infect others. While international efforts have successfully met Millennium Development Goals to reduce new HIV infections overall—especially among infants through PMTCT—HIV incidence is in fact rising among adolescents. AIDS is now the leading cause of death among young people ages ten to nineteen in sub-Saharan Africa (UNICEF 2014).

These adolescents' very survival thus confounds international development narratives by PEPFAR, UNAIDS, UNICEF, and others of creating an "AIDS-free generation." Instead, it has created new forms of anxiety, stigmatization, and marginalization that are as social as they are epidemiological. Bianca Dahl (2012) has investigated how, following Botswana's success in reducing mother-to-child HIV transmission, the continued existence of HIV and AIDS among children extended the stigma of HIV infection, which communities explained through witchcraft, rape, and their parents' moral transgressions (as have PEPFAR's prevention campaigns). Public health messages encouraging testing and treatment for HIV may thus have inadvertently foreclosed more sympathetic interpretations of the illness that might have reduced HIV/AIDS stigma: although people are encouraged to disclose their status in efforts to reduce stigma, many feel it is not worth the risk (Moyer 2012). Caregivers for children and adolescents with HIV also find it challenging to break the news to those children, and so many are coming of age without even realizing their own HIV status (UNICEF 2014)—an issue I examine in more detail in chapter 6, "Suffering, Silence, and Status," through the stories of several HIV-positive children and their caregivers.

Rather than account for the ways that the international AIDS community may have overlooked this age group, the discourse of blame often reverts back to individual behavior. Adolescents pose a challenge to the ongoing fight against HIV/AIDS because of their failure to internalize the unrealistic messages of anti-HIV campaigns—abstinence-only prevention messages, seeking voluntary testing and treatment—and not to the inappropriateness or unfeasibility of the messages themselves. Such emphasis on individual behavior change obfuscates broader political issues that promote the continuance of inequality—age-based or otherwise. Chapter 2 therefore examines the politics of targeting AIDS orphans for humanitarian intervention—against which the choices of young people and their caregivers play out. Though this was to be the first AIDS-free generation, today's young people could well end up in many of the same struggles as the previous generation for prevention, treatment, and social acceptance. So while they are certainly a post-ARV generation, it is premature to label them an AIDS-free generation.

Orphanhood and the Conundrum of
Humanitarian Intervention

If you visit any primary school in Uganda today, you will not be hard-pressed to find an OVC Club there. OVC, short for "orphans and vulnerable children," is one of many acronyms created by the aid and development industries to identify children as targets for programming. Those targets themselves have now come to identify with the categorization to the point where primary schools have clubs for children who once, not long ago, were highly marginalized by the fact of orphanhood. If you visit a primary school OVC Club, you will find that many of the children who are members belong to the club not because they are orphans, consider themselves vulnerable, or even want to stand in solidarity with their orphaned friends; rather, they may explain, as children often did to me, "I joined the OVC Club because sometimes we can get out of classes to go to marches and other stuff." When I was discussing this phenomenon with Dorothy Oulanyah, UNICEF (United Nations Children's Fund, originally the United Nations International Children's Emergency Fund) HIV specialist for OVC prevention in Uganda in 2009, she linked it back to the expansion of the definition of *child vulnerability* by organizations such as her own, pointing out, "It raises very fundamental questions: what exactly are we [achieving by] responding in this way?"[1]

In this chapter, I aim to address this question by detailing the evolution of the global and national response to AIDS orphanhood and its unintended consequences. Many scholars have pointed out the humanitarian appeal of children to the West and problematized development's role in the targeting of children through hegemonic Western constructs of childhood to further neocolonial attitudes that infantilize entire nations (see, e.g., Fassin 2013; Pupavac 2001; Suski 2009; Valentin and Meinert 2009). This type of engagement is enduring and has particular effects that impact children's lives, positively or negatively. In this chapter I therefore draw on critical humanitarian studies, which consider "humanitarian engagement as it is lived" (Bornstein 2012, 19), to examine the effects of OVC targeting more closely, starting with the construction of the category of *orphan* and its evolution in international development context. Exploring the dynamics of childhood vulnerability in the Ugandan context from policy to practice, I further detail the complexities of the development and cultural translation of the definition of *orphans and vulnerable children*, a catch-all phrase developed in the aid industry to recognize the vulnerabilities faced not only by orphans but also by other children lacking care. This process of defining targets gave governments the chance to incorporate lessons learned from NGOs on the frontlines of the "orphan crisis," but the targeting of children in development aid comes with some adverse consequences. Though Ugandans' growing acknowledgement of child vulnerability is in itself seen as an achievement by policy makers, I argue here that OVC targeting has reified vulnerability as an ironically privileged and empowered identity; orphanhood can ironically *raise* the status of a child who has lost a parent precisely because orphans are made objects for intervention. But the expanded definition of OVC imposes a hierarchy of vulnerability that helps determine which of Uganda's estimated 7.5 million OVC will receive assistance. In the midst of ever-dwindling aid resources, children and families in need must adjust strategies to meet the criteria for vulnerability that might gain them access to such resources and create an untenable demand for orphan services—often at the expense of other vulnerable children and communities.

Global to Local Understandings of the Orphan Experience: Expanding Definitions of Vulnerability

Recent scholarship on the entanglements of transnational development regimes with local African AIDS orphans suggests a profound reification of the category *orphan* (Chirwa 2002; Henderson 2006; Meintjes and Giese 2006). As noted in the introduction, policy attention to orphans was largely an afterthought of AIDS policy, once it became clear that orphanhood was a major social aftereffect of the disease that was overburdening traditional systems of care. The Ugandan government's response to mass orphanhood did not come until 2004—twelve years after peak HIV prevalence in 1992—with the rollout of a national OVC policy. However, it should be noted that the humanitarian attention that shifted to orphans in Africa followed not just the trajectory of the AIDS pandemic but also the international campaign for children's rights in the last decade of the twentieth century and the first decade of the twenty-first. A children's rights agenda consequently dominates international OVC policy. The United Nations Convention on the Rights of the Child (CRC), which was adopted in 1989, makes no specific mention—and therefore sets no definition—of orphans.[2] However, UNICEF, anticipating an "orphan crisis" due to AIDS, made a conscious political decision in the late 1990s to define an orphan as "a child under 18 years of age whose mother, father, or both parents have died" (UNICEF 2006, 4). By this definition, an estimated 53 million sub-Saharan African children had been orphaned—30 percent (15.7 million) of them by AIDS—by 2006 (UNICEF 2006, iv). This number has since reduced over the duration of this study, with UNAIDS putting the number of African AIDS orphans at 10.5 million in 2013 due largely to steep declines (more than 50 percent) in AIDS-related mortality in several key African countries from 2005 to 2011 (UNAIDS 2013, 7–8). Uganda's orphan population in 2006 was about two million, or 19 percent of all children in the country (Oleke et al. 2006, 267), and almost half of those children were made orphans due to AIDS (UNICEF 2006). However, UNAIDS estimated that the number of Ugandan children orphaned due to AIDS remained at about 1.1 million in 2013 (UNAIDS 2013, 101).

It should be noted, though, that African vernacular languages rarely have words that mean what *orphan* does in international development parlance. Vernacular terms that most closely translate into *orphan* mean something like "left behind or abandoned" (Chirwa 2002, 96), which is rare compared to children who lose one parent but still have family care. The United Nations (UN) definition thus distorts local definitions and inflates orphan numbers by statically singling out the "orphaned" child as particularly vulnerable despite widespread extended-family social safety nets (Meintjes and Giese 2006). As in many African societies, local definitions of orphanhood in Uganda have historically been based on social delineations, in which situations of actual care are emphasized over the existence of a biological parent. Due to a strong ethos of kin care for children who lose their parents (elaborated on in part 4 of this volume), Ugandan vernacular languages also use terminology to describe orphans by circumstance; children typically have to lose not only their mother and father but also most of their aunts, uncles, and grandparents—and become essentially homeless—to be considered "orphans." The use of Luganda terms for orphans—*mulekwa* and *enfunzi*, for example—are so rare and stigmatizing that my twenty-three-year-old research assistant, whose first language is Luganda, had never heard some of them.

This discrepancy is not unknown to national policy makers, either. Manager of the Uganda OVC National Implementation Unit John Okiror told me in 2009 that the Ateso word for *orphan*, *ekokit*, means "a child who has lost both parents," but Oulanyah noted that "even then, there are many children who would not consider themselves as orphans because either their father's brother is living or their mother's sister is alive."[3]

By contrast, UNICEF's interpretation of orphanhood emphasizes static, biological definitions of kinship and orphanhood in contexts where traditionally, orphans are socially defined within a broad and pliable kin care network. In efforts to raise their visibility, international nongovernmental organizations (NGOs) have highlighted the plight of Africa's AIDS orphans, sometimes at the expense of other children who may have similar or greater needs (Foster, Levine, and Williamson 2005, 3). Further, by focusing on orphans themselves, aid efforts can easily label them in reifying ways that ignore their roles in households, families, communities, and even generations. Thus, rather than emphasizing individual and community resilience, this reification creates an orphan identity that is both pathologized (Henderson 2006, 304) and made a privileged site for benevolent humanitarian intervention (A. Ferguson and Freidus 2007). This intervention often comes with adverse consequences, intended or unintended. For example, such targeting may cause household conflicts over resources and alter community priorities (Foster, Levine, and Williamson 2005, 3). These adverse consequences came about as a result of a conscious choice on the part of UNICEF to highlight the plight of AIDS orphans in anticipation of an "AIDS orphan crisis" in the 1990s. Though this crisis never really came to pass—perhaps because of UNICEF's sounding of the alarm—the expansive definition and its corollary categorizations have had important implications for humanitarian and development targeting of children.

As if to exacerbate the overwhelming statistics generated by the UN definition of *orphan*, the aid industry has also cultivated the terms *orphans and vulnerable children* (OVC) and *children affected by AIDS* (CABA) to emphasize childhood vulnerability generated by the disease. Orphanhood makes children "vulnerable," but NGO field-workers trying to implement orphan policy recognized that other HIV/AIDS–related vulnerabilities based on multiple structural factors were equal if not larger factors in children's vulnerability. For example, deepening poverty due to HIV/AIDS was often a greater issue than orphanhood itself. Further, studies throughout Africa were showing that children are affected by AIDS well before parents die, so interventions for "orphans" often came too late to mitigate vulnerability (Robson and Ansell 2000). In response to the challenges of trying to program specifically for HIV/AIDS–affected orphans, aid organizations began to consider widening the scope of childhood vulnerability due to HIV/AIDS beyond orphanhood. The acronym *OVC* thus evolved within the aid industry to encompass a broader range of children at risk or in difficult circumstances. The heightened level of vulnerability is variously attributed to global economic downturn, the ways fostering households are affected by taking in orphans in crisis, elderly grandparents becoming primary caretakers of both their dying children and their young grandchildren, and particular dimensions of rural/urban poverty. Employing the term *OVC* allowed NGOs to consider their work from broader social development, child protection, and children's rights mandates. This designation also acknowledged that orphans, depending on their circumstances, may not be in as precarious a position as certain other children who still have their parents. Such terms thus help recognize that children other than orphans—even those orphaned by AIDS—are in need of assistance. As for CABA, "Children are affected when their close or extended family, their community, and, more broadly, the structures and services that exist for their benefit are strained by the consequences of the HIV/AIDS pandemic" (Gruskin and Tarantola 2005, 138). However, by this broad definition, practically every child in sub-Saharan Africa is now one of the CABA. This evolution of definitions (see fig. 2) did little to demystify the category of "orphans" as targets for charitable interventions, however, and may in fact have inadvertently set a precedent for more recent waves of orphan rescue culminating in a perverse "orphan addiction" that I return to describe in chapter 8.

Defining Orphans

'Orphan' → OVC → 'Orphan Crisis' → 'Orphan Rescue' → 'Orphan Addiction'

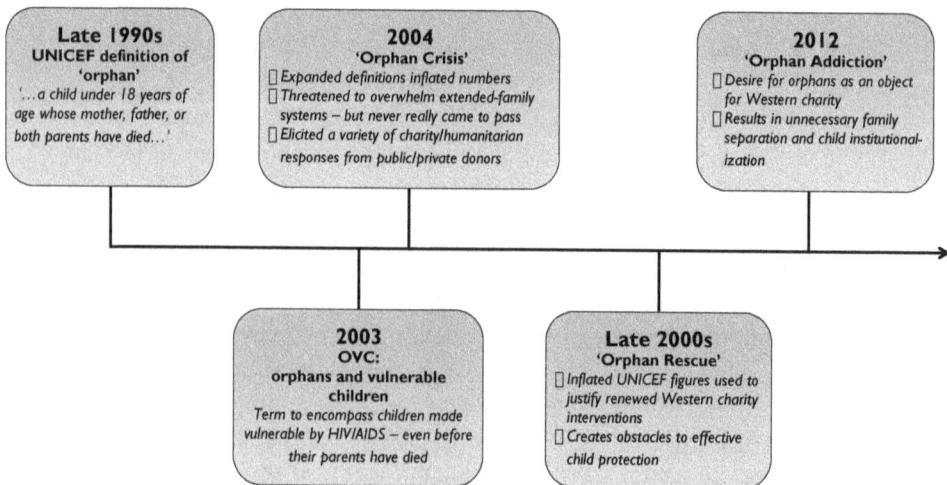

Late 1990s
UNICEF definition of 'orphan'
'...a child under 18 years of age whose mother, father, or both parents have died...'

2004
'Orphan Crisis'
☐ Expanded definitions inflated numbers
☐ Threatened to overwhelm extended-family systems – but never really came to pass
☐ Elicited a variety of charity/humanitarian responses from public/private donors

2012
'Orphan Addiction'
☐ Desire for orphans as an object for Western charity
☐ Results in unnecessary family separation and child institutionalization

2003
OVC:
orphans and vulnerable children
Term to encompass children made vulnerable by HIV/AIDS – even before their parents have died

Late 2000s
'Orphan Rescue'
☐ Inflated UNICEF figures used to justify renewed Western charity interventions
☐ Creates obstacles to effective child protection

FIGURE 2. Time line defining *orphan*: evolution of terms and their consequences.

The Ugandan national OVC policy (Uganda Ministry of Gender, Labour, and Social Development 2004, 2) defines childhood vulnerability as follows:

[A child who is] vulnerable because of any or all of the following factors that result from HIV/AIDS:

- Is HIV-positive
- Lives without adequate adult support (e.g., in a household with chronically ill parents, a household that has experienced a recent death from chronic illness, a household headed by a grandparent, and/or a household headed by a child)
- Lives outside of family care (e.g., in residential care or on the streets), or
- Is marginalized, stigmatized, or discriminated against.

In the spirit of decentralization, the policy goes on to state that "each community will need to prioritize those children most vulnerable and in need of further care" (Uganda Ministry of Gender Labor and Social Development 2004, 2). This leads one to wonder, as Oulanyah did, what in fact such broad targeting actually achieves—especially as the notion of vulnerability becomes increasingly delinked from HIV/AIDS. "It seems we are at a point as a country where we are saying the vulnerability due to HIV and AIDS is actually no different from the vulnerability due to other causes," Oulanyah told me in 2009, "so we are kind of in that process of transitioning from focusing on vulnerability due to HIV and AIDS to vulnerability in general." While recognition of children's multiple vulnerabilities is important, it again inflates the population of children targeted for (largely nonexistent) services. Oulanyah estimated that policy definitions of childhood vulnerability described approximately 70 percent of the nation's children.[4] Though such a model of child vulnerability is not necessarily inaccurate for many of Africa's children, the Ugandan government's growing acknowledgement of child vulnerability is in itself seen as an achievement by children's rights advocates even while it creates an untenable demand for OVC services.

Nonetheless, Oulanyah also worked closely with another UNICEF program called Protecting the Vulnerable (PTV), where they often talked about the interrelatedness of vulnerabilities to avoid limiting their approach. The name Protecting the Vulnerable came from a clause of the UN Millennium Declaration that focused on international humanitarian and human rights law, recognizing that "children and all civilian populations . . . suffer disproportionately the consequences of natural disasters, genocide, armed conflicts and other humanitarian emergencies" (United Nations 2000, 7). Africa was also singled out in the Millennium Declaration, given that it was the world's only region to become poorer in the 1990s (United Nations 2000).

While Africa saw some improvements, an interim report predicted that the continent would fall short of most 2015 Millennium Development Goals (MDG); while there were significant reductions in AIDS-related deaths—including the prevention of infant infection through aggressive PMTCT—other AIDS-related goals in relation to children and youth remained unmet (UNICEF 2014). UNICEF consequently created the PTV program within its various country offices to focus on implementation of that particular MDG provision.

Now the same type of expansion that occurred with the definition of *orphan* is happening with the category of "vulnerable children," though this time the widening of the target population means that the numbers of vulnerable children are much, much higher—and thus create even more untenable demands on public funds. *Vulnerability* is now variously used in Africa to define children as objects for developmental and humanitarian intervention, often in problematic and contrary ways. When I first visited Oulanyah at UNICEF in March 2009, she and her colleagues were working in conjunction with the Uganda Bureau of Statistics to determine the number of orphans and vulnerable children in the country. "It's amazing how creative we can be, categorizing the vulnerabilities!" Oulanyah laughed. Oulanyah pointed out that "for the doctors as long as you are not immunized you are very vulnerable, so count all those who are not immunized. For education, as long as you have dropped out of school you are vulnerable. . . . So how are we going to produce a report that really tells the President that 90-something percent of the children in your country are vulnerable!?" The numbers of children who fall under the OVC policy's purview do indeed range from 50 to 90 percent of the child population, depending on who is counting: within a few months, a USAID official told me that there were 7 million vulnerable children, 2 million of them orphans, and 1 million of those AIDS orphans; and the Uganda Ministry of Gender, Labour, and Social Development (2013) claimed that of the 7.5 million vulnerable children in Uganda, 2.3 million of them were orphans, whereas UNICEF (2013) reported that in 2011 there were 2.6 million orphans, 1.1 million of them by AIDS.

It may sound convoluted, but statistics are an inextricable technology of the international aid industry. "If you don't have criteria," Oulanyah pointed out, "how are you going to know whom it is you are going to reach?" Yet, in reality, the criteria became far too diffuse, especially in an aid industry that favors selective targeting over broader poverty-reduction efforts. Vulnerabilities due to HIV/AIDS are still those that receive greatest priority because they can be linked to funding. According to Herbert Mugumya, senior OVC technical adviser of USAID in 2009, orphan assistance programs usually have to piggyback on HIV/AIDS programs because that is where the money is. So the transition away from HIV/AIDS–based vulnerability is still incomplete, but many of the same mistakes are being replicated: Okiror claimed that translating *vulnerable children* into vernacular languages is even harder than translating *orphan* because there is not typically a simple term for it. As a result, people are locally adopting the English terminology to signal their compatibility with the conditions that would entitle them to services, a point I will return to later in this chapter. Thus, as the attention to the "AIDS orphan crisis" precipitated a whole set of contradictory implications for aid, so now does the expansion of the notion of childhood vulnerability.

Vulnerability, Neoliberalism, and Development

While anthropologists have been studying international development since the discipline's birth in colonial Africa (Falk Moore 1994; Schumaker 2001), they have just recently begun to embrace the study of children as social agents in their own right (James, Jenks, and Prout 1998). Studies of children and national development are rarely linked in anthropology (Cheney 2007b), despite the pervasive targeting of children by global aid, charity, and development campaigns (R. Mahon 2010).

Critical humanitarian studies (Bornstein and Redfield 2010; Feldman and Ticktin 2010) consider how, in Fassin's words, "hierarchies of humanity are passively established but rarely identified for what they are—politics of life that at moments of crisis, result in the formation of two groups, those whose status protects their sacred character and those whom the institutions may sacrifice against their will" (Fassin 2007a, 516). As studies of the cultural meanings of childhood have shown, children definitely fall into the former category of the protected and sacred. My aim here is thus to bring critical humanitarian studies into conversation with children and youth studies to consider the ways that childhood is depoliticized in the aid industry, despite the fact that both domains are rife with politics (Malkki 2010). African children especially are commonly made objects of aid agendas, local and global, to mask political agendas (Fassin 2013). It is exactly when global neoliberal regimes deploy childhood through aid that humanitarianism takes on the air not of a right or entitlement but of a *gift* to blamelessly vulnerable others (Bornstein 2012). Lilie Chouliaraki therefore concludes that "despite . . . its benign objectives of maximizing efficiency and increasing accountability to donors, the financial regime of the aid and development field ultimately legitimizes a neoliberal logic of governance that turns the cosmopolitan aspirations of humanitarianism into the corporate aspirations of the West and, in doing so, not only fails to serve the ideal of global civil society but delivers harmful effects on vulnerable others" (2013, 7).

Vulnerability is often—but not always—conceptually tied to poverty. It is not incidental, then, that the proliferation of the concept of vulnerability closely follows the trajectory of global neoliberal economic policies developed by the International Monetary Fund and the World Bank. Despite promises that "deregulation and privatization would prove a panacea for African economic stagnation" (J. Ferguson 2006, 11), structural adjustment programs (SAPs) only increased economic hardship and inequality through cuts to social welfare that disproportionately affected children. The presumption was that wealth generated at the top of such uneven growth would trickle down. Yet neoliberal policies prevailed in the post-SAP era, in the form of nongovernmental organizations. The growth of NGOs in the late 1980s and early 1990s was largely based on a neoliberal democratization agenda that held that working through unfettered markets allowed more grassroots participation and empowerment, especially when targeting particularly vulnerable populations (Fisher 1997); hence the recent popularity of microcredit programs and donor support for strengthening civil society by redirecting funding from presumably corrupted states to local and international NGOs that "were understood as more 'direct' or 'grassroots' channels of implementation" (J. Ferguson 2006, 38), a sort of populist privatization of care provisioning.

Though some scholars claim that more powerful NGOs contribute to quality service delivery when left to pursue their own agendas (Michael 2004), critics of the proliferation of NGOs contend that NGOs depoliticize the structural roots of poverty by focusing on vulnerable populations rather than transforming the structures (and structural violence) that give rise to their vulnerability. Further, this depoliticization suggests that NGO operations, especially those focusing on children, are somehow apolitical when in fact they are highly politicized arenas (J. Ferguson 1994; Cheney 2007b 12–13). Instead, governments were "decapacitated" by the redirection of donor funds to NGOs (J. Ferguson 2006, 38). In addition, the conflation of democracy and "freedom" with free markets has obfuscated the power relations that uphold poverty and that bear "uncanny similarities to the late-colonial orders of exclusion and exploitation" (Englund 2006, 200).

In Uganda, this conflation takes shape in the form of, among other things, support of the arguably benevolent dictatorship of Yoweri Museveni, whose lengthy rule began when he seized power in 1986 and was most recently extended in February 2016 when he was declared the winner of yet another highly controversial presidential election marred with irregularities (Karimi, Ntale, and Botelho 2016; Winsor 2016), as well as the privatization of industry and migration of qualified staff from government to NGOs (Seeley 2014, 58; Whyte 2014, 8). Overall growth alongside deepening income inequality and (child) poverty, exacerbated by AIDS deaths and the consequent dissolution of households, has led to the selling of land assets in rural areas, where "credit often still derives mainly from family and friends" (Seeley 2014, 59). Child vulnerability cannot be extricated from these broader developments.

BENEVOLENT INTERVENTIONS
FOR VULNERABLE CHILDREN

Children are not exempt from neoliberalism's deleterious effects. Jennifer Cole and Deborah Durham assert that "the current climate of economic liberalization has plunged children into the center of the market in ways that previous laws sought to prevent. The processes associated with globalization —be they socially progressive or neoliberal—challenge older ways of constructing childhood" (2008, 16–17). In the current political economic climate, African children are increasingly being constructed as victims in need of "rescue." This construction of childhood vulnerability fits well with the neoliberal configuration of global capital, perhaps because the kinds of humanitarianism for children produced by NGOs are also well suited to the neoliberal state, which is then off the hook for providing services to needy populations (A. Ferguson and Freidus 2007). These kinds of humanitarianism also appeal to the desires of Western donors to "save" the needy children of the global South. Recognized members of vulnerable childhood identities—orphan, child soldier, street child—thereby become a means to make claims, or tap the market of available aid to vulnerable children.

Terence Ranger in his edited volume *Evangelical Christianity and Democracy in Africa* (2008) has discussed the gradual conjoining of evangelical Christianity with democratic movements in Africa since the anticolonial independence movements of the twentieth century. The discourse of Christian faith-based humanitarian initiatives share much with free-market ideologies. As Erica Bornstein notes, "The construction of individuals in relation to the divine, as conceived of by the Christian discourse of faith-based NGOs, parallels neoliberal assumptions of individual 'choice' that underlie the discourse of a 'free-market'"(2003, 5). Although churches and faith-based organizations have a long history of assisting orphans, children are similarly made objects of intervention by a humanitarian industry that is often undergirded by neoconservative, evangelical ideology. This trend toward "compassionate conservatism" is exemplified by recent US foreign policy. Programs such as PEPFAR have followed neoliberal economic policies and neoconservative social agendas. For example, just before founding PEPFAR, the George W. Bush administration revoked US funding for the United Nations Population Fund (UNFPA, the abbreviation retained from its original name, United Nations Fund for Population Activities) and in 2001 reinstated the global abortion gag rule, which prohibits US funding to any NGO conducting family planning (Barot and Cohen 2015). Indeed, pro-nat(ion)alist policies under both government and international NGOs during this early twenty-first-century period are at least partly a function of capitalist discourses of productivist expansion. At the same time as they championed programs for children, though, such policies contributed to overpopulation, maternal mortality, and rising rates of new HIV infection. While neoliberal policies drive the supposedly benevolent humanitarianism that would target vulnerable populations with services, the accompanying rise in population continues to deepen poverty by putting undue strain on limited natural resources—most important, food and land. Focusing on enumerating the numbers of individual vulnerable children in this context thus belies the bigger issues of poverty and structural violence that affect entire populations. Leslie Butt calls this the trope of "the suffering stranger," which "is primarily the result of the imperative to try to speak for others on a global front. The use of truncated tales of suffering strangers prioritizes international moralities over local experiences" (2002, 3).

Under this construction, children deserve intervention precisely because they are considered voiceless and innocent, thrust into circumstances not of their choosing. It is important to consider the tensions this scenario raises—namely, whether defining vulnerability also generates vulnerability. By taking humanitarianism as the social field of analysis, we can assess the process through which categories of vulnerability are globally and locally reproduced and examine their impacts on children. Having laid out for consideration the ways in which vulnerability has been constructed to create avenues of global humanitarian assistance for children in Africa, I turn to the consequences for a nation that has ever fewer resources with which to reach the children who fall under vulnerability's widening umbrella. How has this expansion of the definition of *vulnerability* strayed from its intended outcomes? Some of the vagueness of the concept is exploited, I suggest, not only by donors and state agencies wishing to further their own agendas but also by children and their guardians.

ADVERSE CONSEQUENCES OF ORPHAN TARGETING

When African governments and the international aid industry recognized the proliferation of orphans and childhood vulnerability due to AIDS, and indeed defined it as a "crisis," they targeted orphans problematically, with un-intended consequences. As detailed in part 4, extended family is usually the first line of response when a child in Africa loses his or her parents, and there is a long history of fosterage, well documented in anthropological literature, that has served to mitigate many social stresses before the AIDS pandemic in Africa. After the proliferation of orphans due to AIDS—and the death of aunts and uncles as well as mothers and fathers—stretched the capacity of many extended family networks beyond their limits (Aspaas 1999; Oleke, Blystad, and Rekdal 2005), NGOs stepped in to help; however, they did so in ways that not only disrupted African traditions of fosterage but also trans-formed local categories of childhood vulnerability.

One local NGO learned early on what happens when organizations target orphans exclusively for assistance. Uganda Women's Effort to Save Orphans (UWESO) was founded by Uganda's first lady, Janet Museveni, in 1986 to assist war orphans in the wake of the civil war that brought her husband to power. As the needs of war orphans waned and the AIDS pandemic started leaving more and more children orphaned, UWESO was in a unique position to shift its focus to AIDS orphans. By then, it had also learned a few lessons about the politics of orphan assistance. UWESO projects coordinator Baker Waiswa explained to me that they started out paying school fees for orphans—almost all of whom were cared for by extended family. But they quickly observed that, whereas orphans' status within extended family households started out rather low, UWESO's direct assistance to orphans actually raised their sta-tus above that of other household members. "The families were so poor," he said, "that the [sponsored] orphans went to school and the biological children sometimes failed to go to school. So it even posed a challenge to the parents. You cannot explain to a child and say, 'Yes, I love you, though I am not able to take you to school.' [Children will] say, 'But what about this one??' However much you explain, 'Well, they brought money, etc.' they kind of can't believe it, so it was a problem."[5]

UWESO knew then that targeting orphans alone was not sustainable and caused too much tension in the families. Aside from creating inequali-ties within the household, UWESO also had guardians relinquishing their responsibilities for orphans on the assumption that UWESO had replaced them: guardians would even stop coming to visit orphans at boarding schools on visiting days. When UWESO approached the guardians and asked why they did not visit their children, they would say, rather perplexed, "They're UWESO's children now."[6] UWESO has therefore ended direct educational assistance and instead offers income generation assistance to households with orphans, so that all children—and guardians—in the household stand to benefit. UWESO prioritizes them in terms of their level of vulnerability: child-headed households are the first priority, followed by grandparent-headed households, and those taking care of many children (they found one grandparent taking care of twenty-three grandchildren).

Guardians who were part of this study were clearly aware that OVC identity had become commoditized as NGOs targeted them for assistance. As mentioned at the beginning of this chapter, vernacular terms such as *mulekwa* in Luganda carry meanings that translate roughly as "one who is abandoned or left with no one." The stigma attached to vernacular terms indicates that they are not words to be used lightly or liberally, especially in the presence of children to whom they might apply, because they would be made to feel marginalized and pitied. Such terms are thus wielded with extreme caution in local social contexts. Not so with English: while people may hesitate to label children by a comparable vernacular term, claiming to be an "orphan" becomes an ironically privileged and empowered identity when donors and NGOs target such children for assistance. Now, where guardians would still not dare call a child *mulekwa* in his or her presence, they gladly parade their "orphans" (in English, the language of international aid) before potential benefactors. This is because presenting as an "orphan," in international aid parlance, may now literally pay. Some guardians therefore consciously cultivate an OVC identity in children, coaching them to emphasize their material deprivation in order to solicit handouts. Even when two children in my study died, the family brought two more to "replace" them on the assumption that assistance would be forthcoming for children in the study (though we had tried to be clear with guardians that it would not). I even had to drop one family from the study because their grandmother had trained the grandchildren she was caring for to detail their material deprivations in the absence of their parents, and their responses to our questions were so scripted that we felt that—for the integrity of our research and for their own well-being—we could not include them. The intervention of international aid on behalf of children orphaned by AIDS has thus not only reified OVC and complicated family relationships by introducing incentives to orphans and family members willing to take them in but has cultivated a positive identification with vulnerability. Oulanyah saw a similar effect in UNICEF programming when children they served started wishing their parents dead; she told me, "We've got children who actually say, 'Well, if *my* mom and dad died, maybe *I* could get schoolbooks.'"[7]

Despite the lessons learned, there has been a proliferation of international NGOs that have made orphans their exclusive objects of assistance, and plenty of them are replicating the pattern of prioritizing orphans over other needy children as well as reifying the orphan from family and community. In this way, the rhetoric of vulnerability continues to trickle down into the operational language of NGOs, which want to show that they share the same commitments to helping OVC, as well as families and communities who hope to gain by connecting their "orphans" to services that are otherwise not accessible.

VULNERABILITY'S BENEFICIARIES

If categories such as OVC have such adverse effects, why use them at all? If poverty is the root problem, why not just extend services to all children and enumerate specific qualifications instead of creating such problematic identifications? Are these categorizations even avoidable? Perhaps the state means to create these ineffable categories because it too hopes to gain: given that the Ugandan government budget is typically comprised of more than 50 percent donor funding, identifying "90-something percent" of children as vulnerable could mean that the government could claim even more donor funding for OVC programming. The appeal, by government or individuals, is to donors' and NGOs' sense of charity toward children and not actually to expanding state services that would serve OVC, as funds rarely leave the ministry offices, let alone reach those whom they are meant to assist. On the other hand, by creating a national OVC policy without a service delivery budget, the government gains more oversight of the local and international NGOs that might have otherwise flown under their radar, thereby reclaiming some control of the humanitarian capital going toward AIDS-affected children. According to Helen Epstein, "Every government ministry, from Education to Labor to Defense, now has an AIDS budget" (2007, 206). In 2009, the former director of the Uganda Center for Accountability, Teddy Cheeye, was convicted of embezzling 120 million Uganda shillings (about 56,000 US dollars) from the Global Fund to Fight AIDS, Tuberculosis and Malaria (Wandera 2009). Such misappropriation is grave and explicit, but with corruption at every level from national to household, funds can be skimmed until nothing is left (Scherz 2014, 57). Further, the allocation of aid resources has more subtle stakes: under Bush's PEPFAR plan, faith-based organizations with no experience in AIDS prevention were eligible to receive PEPFAR money and have been using it to further a neoconservative social agenda that emphasizes, among other things, abstinence-only education (Human Rights Watch/ Africa 2005). Under pressure from donors and religious groups, President Museveni reversed his position on the ABC approach (abstinence, be faithful, use condoms) to HIV prevention and started promoting abstinence only. As a result, new HIV infections in the 2010s have begun to rise for the first time since the 1990s.[8]

The most unfortunate consequence, however, is not the exploitation of OVC and other AIDS-affected people but that adhering to hegemonic notions of vulnerability perpetuated in aid discourse and practice reinstates not only the victimhood of children but also the neocolonial representation of Africa as a continent perpetually in need of assistance from outside sources, whether they be foreign government donors or international aid organizations. So while it remains a purposefully vague notion, vulnerability is being fully instrumentalized, creating hierarchies of need by those who define it.

The influence of aid for OVC on the dynamics of extended-family care is apparent in the ways that families make decisions about how to allocate caregiving responsibilities for orphans after their parents have died. Orphans are typically reared by relatives of their extended family, who in the past rarely received material assistance from sources outside the family. While several scholars have detailed a long African tradition of child circulation and fosterage for adult self-interest (Bledsoe and Isiugo-Abanihe 1989; Notermans 2004), Oleke and colleagues note "a transition over the past 30 years from a situation dominated by 'Purposeful' voluntary exchange of non-orphaned children to one dominated by 'crisis fostering' of orphans" (Oleke, Blystad, and Rekdal 2005, 2628). But in a state of general lack of resources, the introduction of funding targeted specifically at caregivers of orphans can provide extra incentives to foster that do not necessarily increase children's well-being. Orphans who turn to their elders for care and support may manipulate the orphans' disenfranchisement for their own material gain (Patterson 2003, 24). For example, UWESO regularly found that when it distributed supplies such as mosquito nets directly to orphans, the caregivers typically commandeered the donations for themselves or their biological children.[9] In a more egregious example, instances of land grabbing—in which relatives of children left orphaned offer to care for them on their parents' property and then chase the children off the property after a month or two—are all too common throughout the continent (Rose 2005). Our study similarly found that family decisions to take in orphans increasingly hinged on what benefits the adults would gain by taking in children rather than the other way around—and considerations of aid entitlement have become significant factors. Of late, foreign assistance for orphans is even becoming a factor in decisions to institutionalize children, as I elaborate in part 4.

With or without assistance, orphans have become commoditized in a chain of local and global support. OVC and their guardians thus tend to appropriate—and even embrace—the tropes of vulnerability placed on them by discourses of benevolent humanitarianism. As I show in later chapters, children's own innovative survival strategies also tend to capitalize on the "vulnerable child" discourse.

As the codifying of OVC identities re-creates orphans as sites for both local and global humanitarian intervention, children and adults alike thus learn how to "work it," manipulating the powerful social categories placed on OVC by both local and global discourses about orphans to procure resources in a resource-strapped environment. For example, Viva, an international orphan advocacy group, did a census of orphan services and found that some families were receiving school fees for the same child from as many as three different organizations.[10]

As I hope to make clear in later chapters, most guardians are sincere and selfless in their efforts to care for children left without parental care. It is nonetheless important to identify these patterns, but interpreting their appropriation of OVC identity as an act of postcolonial mimicry (Young 2003, 141) or fulfilling the "script" of childhood helplessness would be too simplistic. We might instead see OVC and their caregivers as renegotiating the disempowering language of international aid in hopes of gaining entitlement to basic human rights and social justice through the back door: "I am vulnerable, and I therefore have a right to assistance." But this view also plays into the neoliberal hierarchy of humanity (Fassin 2007a), in which children—particularly orphans—are more deserving by virtue of having "done nothing to deserve their poverty." We can discern, in these actions, examples of children's resilience and agentive skills in navigating the adverse conditions of their existence as orphans. The drawback is that their own strategies tend to play into an ethos of charity that defers understanding of children's rights as transformatively empowering rather than simply protectionist—an issue I examine in chapter 3.

PART TWO

Beyond Checking the "Voice" Box: Children's Rights and Participation in Development and Research

3

Children's Rights: Participation, Protectionism, and Citizenship

As mentioned in part 1, at around the same time as the drafting of national policies regarding orphans and vulnerable children (OVC), African government signatories of the Convention on the Rights of the Child (CRC) and nongovernmental organizations (NGOs) were widely adopting rights-based approaches in their OVC programming. According to Save the Children, which started implementing rights-based approaches in 1999, "A rights-based approach to development considers the fulfillment of everyone's human rights as the end goal of development" (Save the Children 2006, 14). The development of rights-based approaches was meant to address the structural issues that needs-based approaches—which are charity-driven rather than policy-driven—do not, making space for the empowerment of development aid's target populations and opening the possibility for societal transformation (Abdelmoneium 2008). However, the concept of empowerment was quickly co-opted by neoliberal institutions that reduced it from a mode of transformative collective action to a "Foucauldian" means of individual self-improvement within market-based national economies (Pease 2002; McEwen and Bek 2006).

Due to the ways aid organizations and government policies have targeted OVC, rights-based approaches have thus far failed to achieve widespread empowerment of children—nor have they adequately addressed the structural causes of the problems of orphans. Instead, the adoption of the CRC as a mandate for aid organizations' humanitarian interventions found expression mainly in the application of the "best interests" principle. According to this principle, adults and adult institutions should make the best interests of children a primary consideration in any activities or policy making that affects children. Like other key concepts in the CRC, however, the term *best interests* was intentionally left undefined by the CRC committee to account for local context and circumstances (Arts 2010, 14). While this intentional vagueness was established with respect for cultural diversity and local specificity in mind, it hinders the actionability of children's rights for OVC because the convergence of the AIDS epidemic, children's rights discourses, and the international development community's intervention in traditional extended-family systems of orphan support triply disenfranchise orphaned children through constant reinstatement of their vulnerability rather than their collective empowerment through rights. Further, attention to the way in which AIDS in particular is made the culprit conceals the vulnerabilities of children (not only orphans) created by the devastation of neoliberal, postcolonial state restructuring and Africa's destabilization by the global free-market economy (Englund 2006). Because children are deprived daily of food security, health care, housing, and education by the vagaries of the free market and Uganda's crippling foreign debt and corruption, children's rights cannot be made meaningful without full acknowledgement of their violation, especially economically and socially. The efforts of international NGOs to address this vulnerability through a discourse of benevolent humanitarianism enshrined in CRC-style protectionism—without directly addressing broader issues of structural poverty through a discourse of human rights—has serious consequences for pursuing children's rights, most especially for "vulnerable" orphans, because of the ways they reproduce tropes of orphan victimhood.

The reasons for this vulnerability can be traced to the ways in which children's rights were conceptualized in the first place. The concept of children's rights arose in the West in the wake of the Industrial Revolution of the late eighteenth and early nineteenth centuries. In the twentieth century, children came to be seen as naturally innocent and precious (Zelizer 1985) but incompetent and vulnerable (World Bank 2005)—and therefore in need of protection.[1] The construction of children's rights was therefore primarily informed by Western developmental psychology's understandings of childhood (James 2011), whose underlying presumptions about children as people in need of protection justified the removal of children not only from the factory but from public space more generally, hypersurveillance of children (Katz 2003), deferred citizenship (Cheney 2007b), and their separation from adults in specialized institutions such as schools (Fass 2008, 34). Children came to be seen as belonging in private space and ensconced in the bosom of the nuclear family. Yet rights discourses contradictorily lift them out of those spaces by granting individual rights that they as rights bearers cannot claim because they need an adult interlocutor to help claim or even fulfill their entitlements. Then they are expected to go to adults or adult institutions for redress when their rights are denied to them. This is the way children's rights are universally codified in, for example, international human rights law.

THE CRC: PARTICIPATORY OR PROTECTIONIST?

One of the routes to empowerment of children is through participation in decisions that affect them. Children's rights scholars and practitioners alike have contended that the CRC is guided by principles of child participation and/or child protection. The website of the United Nations Children's Fund, originally United Nations International Children's Emergency Fund (UNICEF), in describing the CRC states, "Human rights apply to all age groups; children have the same general human rights as adults. But children are particularly vulnerable and so they also have particular rights that recognize their special need for protection" (UNICEF 2005). Indeed, the words *protection* and *protect* occur not less than forty-seven times in the CRC (versus nineteen times in the Universal Declaration of Human Rights), while the African Charter on the Rights and Welfare of the Child (ACRWC) uses the term *protect* thirty-three times. Even the stated purpose of the Ugandan Government's Children Act is "to provide for local authority support for children" (Government of Uganda 1997, 1); it does not contain the word *participation*. Similarly, the terms *empowerment*, *empower*, or even *power* do not appear at all in any of these documents.

Many scholars have endorsed UNICEF's contention that "participation is one of the guiding principles of the [CRC]" (UNICEF n.d.a). However, this seems a broad interpretation when *participation* is not even defined as a key term in the introduction (UNICEF n.d.b), and the word appears only twice in the whole document (as opposed to five appearances in the Universal Declaration of Human Rights): once in Article 23 on disability, where it says that states should facilitate disabled children's active participation in community, and once in Article 40, where it actually refers not to children but to other witnesses in penal cases involving children. Other mentions of children's right to "participate" are in relation to separation from family (Article 9) and play (Article 31). The African Charter on the Rights and Welfare of the Child similarly refers only to participation of disabled children in cultural and leisure activities. Article 12 is often referred to as the main participation provision in the CRC, but it does not use the term *participation*, either. Rather, it states:

1. States Parties shall assure to the child who is capable of forming his or her own views *the right to express those views freely in all matters affecting the child*, the views of the child being given due weight in accordance with the age and maturity of the child.

2. For this purpose, *the child shall in particular be provided the opportunity to be heard* in any judicial and administrative proceedings affecting the child, either directly, or through a representative or an appropriate body, in a manner consistent with the procedural rules of national law. (United Nations 1989, my emphasis)

These provisions are about the expression of views, and not participation in decision making per se. As with *participation*, what it means to *be heard* is open to interpretation. The phrase also appears to refer to individual children and not to entire groups (such as orphans), who are subject to policy implementation. Even UNICEF, in its generous interpretation of the CRC as guaranteeing participation, acknowledges that "expressing an opinion is not the same as taking a decision, but it implies the ability to influence decisions" (UNICEF n.d.b). So Article 12 and other references to children's rights regarding the expression of views is still, at best, a precursor to children as a social group being able to influence decision-making processes and policies that affect them.

This lack of clarity and emphasis on participation in the CRC leaves one to wonder where people got the idea that participation is enshrined in children's rights conventions. Despite no obvious emphasis in the documents, many observers still insist that the CRC itself emphasizes children's participation in decisions that affect them—any discrepancies resting with implementation alone. While a basic content analysis of the CRC indicates that it emphasizes protection over participation, I suspect that the stakes in recognizing participation as a guiding principle of the CRC may be linked to emphases in childhood studies on children's agency. Although it has been fairly well established that children do have both rights and agency (Franklin 1986; Stephens 1995; Jenks 1996; Mayall 1999), attention must now turn to how that agency is constrained under difficult circumstances, such as orphanhood. I argue that the fact that protection and "best interests" are emphasized so much more than participation or empowerment in these documents points to the underlying assumption of children's vulnerability and reliance on adults, and that this assumption is what still informs practice. Take, for instance, the fact that human rights declarations generally allow adults to make direct claims for their rights while children cannot, which makes children's rights different from other human rights from their inception—and perhaps to some extent they should be, as it is important to acknowledge children's age-related developmental distinctiveness by providing more protection (Ennew 2002). On the other hand, implementing children's rights protections requires adult interlocutors to intervene on children's behalf to make claims on their rights

(Brennan 2002). This necessity for adult interlocutors does not necessarily help children to be empowered by rights, then, as children must still rely on adult gatekeepers to take the first agentive steps to fulfill even their basic rights.

Despite this intergenerational dependence, the CRC still refers to "the child" in singular isolation. In 1947, Melville Herskovitz prepared a draft statement on the Universal Declaration of Human Rights for the American Anthropological Association. In it, he expressed concern for the ethos of universal individuality in it:

> It is a truism that groups are composed of individuals, and human beings do not function outside the societies of which they form a part. The problem is thus to formulate a statement of human rights that will do more than just phrase respect for the individual as an individual. It must also take into full account the individual as a member of the social group of which he is a part, whose sanctioned modes of life shape his behavior, and with whose fate his own is thus inextricably bound. (Executive Board of the American Anthropological Association 1947, 539)

Thus began the discipline of anthropology's contentious relationship with human rights, where anthropologists want to uphold human rights while continuing to problematize their very conception. It is surprising, then, when anthropologists of childhood in particular are so keen to uncritically accept the CRC as a guiding document,[2] when the notion of children's rights are arguably even more cross-culturally contested. Similar to Herskovitz's claim that human rights are fundamentally flawed because they are constructed for the individual while people live in cultural groups with diverse notions of individual sovereignty and freedom, so one could argue that children's rights are flawed because they do little to recognize the interrelational and culturally constructed nature of childhood outside of the need for protection. This view simply does not reflect the social reality of most children's lives. Further, the recent development of the field of childhood studies has helped situate the concept of childhood socially and historically, establishing that while childhood as a biological stage is universal, what it means to be a child varies significantly across societies and historical periods (Aries 1962; Alanen 2001; Schwartzman 2001).

The CRC Optional Protocol 3, ratified in February 2012, allows "children the possibility to access justice at the international level through a newly adopted complaints procedure" (Child Rights Coalition Asia 2012). This protocol holds promise for increasing children's participation, but it is still optional. Contradicting UNICEF's claim that "children have the same general human rights as adults," Peter Newell, the chair of the NGO coalition that pushed for the optional protocol said, "It was high time to put children's rights on an equal footing with other human rights! . . . Children's rights are no longer 'mini rights'" (Child Rights International Network [CRIN] 2011). Whether the optional protocol will put children's rights on equal footing with adults' rights remains to be seen, depending on the committee's actions and the implementation of states parties. Although twenty states initially signed the optional protocol, they would not be bound by it until it was actually ratified by at least ten states (Child Rights Coalition Asia 2012). Optional Protocol 3 finally went into force on April 14, 2014, enabling children from those states which have ratified it to bring complaints about rights violations directly to the UN Committee on the Rights of the Child. However, because the violation must have taken place after April 14, 2014, and national mechanisms for addressing such children's rights violations must first be exhausted before the UN Committee will hear them, it could be some time before a complaint reaches them (Child Rights Connect 2014). As of May 2, 2016, Optional Protocol 3 had twenty-eight signatories and twenty-seven states parties (United Nations Human Rights Office of the High Commissioner 2016).

THE RELATIONSHIP BETWEEN
RIGHTS AND VULNERABILITY

We have seen that, despite its broad applications, labeling children as "vulnerable" is meant to give rise to agency among them and their families by opening avenues to entitlement. Under a truly rights-based approach, this might be advantageous, but given the CRC's protectionist approach in practice, children themselves, rather than ineffectively trying to claim their rights, are embracing their orphanhood and vulnerability to secure the resources of charitable organizations.

In the introduction, I described an encounter with a child named Margaret, who went soliciting educational support immediately upon the death of her guardian. I could not possibly meet all the many verbal and written requests I received, from guardians and children, for educational sponsorship of orphans, so I explained to her that I was a student without many means. I suggested that she seek assistance from one of the NGOs whose offices were ubiquitous in the city of Kampala. Had she tried any of the NGOs in town to see about educational assistance? In a 2008 survey, Viva International found more than five hundred organizations in Kampala working on OVC issues,[3] so there was certainly no shortage. She answered that she had gone to Christian Children's Fund, but they had essentially slammed the door in her face, telling her she would need to come back with an adult to vouch for her. The point was that with the death of her uncle, she was left with fewer and fewer possible adult interlocutors. But she could hardly go knock on the door of the Ministry of Education to demand her right to go to school, either, so she had come to Christian Children's Fund to seek assistance.

Even as narratives of vulnerability tend to reify orphans, stories like Margaret's demonstrate how children's abilities to act on their own behalf are still thwarted by systems of power that emphasize protectionist discourses of children's rights instead of participatory ones. If all rights claims necessarily require access to a public sphere that is not so much a space of rational deliberation as a site of power (Asad 2003, 184), orphans' vulnerabilities in particular reveal how little access children actually have to their rights. Advocacy groups turn out to be a necessary intermediary in the process to claiming rights, yet children cannot even access those groups without a guardian's assistance.

This lack of accessibility does not stop children like Margaret from trying to secure NGO resources for themselves, though. Children who learn about children's rights—through schools or through government or NGO "sensitization" campaigns—may utilize the language of rights to try to operationalize them in their own interests, but such children are quickly dissuaded of the tactic by the very institutions that promote children's rights (such as schools) as these institutions often stress obedience to adults over assertion of rights (Cheney 2007b, 66–69).

THE DISEMPOWERING ROLE OF CHILDREN'S RIGHTS

In sum, the way children's rights have been operationalized, particularly in relation to OVC, is incommensurate with thinking of children as rights bearers because it strips them of their capacity to make claims on their rights. While many aid organizations have shifted to rights-based approaches, these constructions of orphans as particularly vulnerable lead the aid industry to continue to emphasize protectionist aspects of children's rights discourse rather than children's empowerment through rights. Children's rights can thus reproduce the status quo between children and adults, in part due to their Western conceptualization as described earlier in the chapter. Addressing children as part of nuclear households as well as extended-family networks is not the problem per se; children can act as rights bearers within the family. And children are indeed vulnerable beings, but history shows that this is a social designation as much as a natural one. This hegemonic notion of childhood reinforces the imperative of all adults to act as duty bearers—even in children's rights–based approaches. Combine this imperative with the neo-liberal influence that has led to the privatization of development in the hands of civil society rather than government, and making claims on the state as the ultimate duty bearer of rights to its citizens becomes even more difficult as services become more market-based and commercialized to appeal to private donors. The responsibility for survival and social reproduction is passed on to the individual. So what happens to OVC like Margaret, when there is no one else left to vouch that they are deserving of even charity, let alone rights?

Starting instead with the perceived needs of children conjures up Maslow's hierarchy and in that regard might be seen as working toward the fulfillment of rights; some scholars will claim that basic needs must often be met before rights can be fulfilled. Judith Ennew refers to the "three P's" of the CRC—provision, protection, and participation—suggesting that they also constitute a kind of hierarchy in which the first takes priority and the rest are achieved sequentially (Ennew 2002). Because of the ways rights-based approaches have been conceptualized and implemented in OVC programming, however, none are adequately fulfilled, which raises the question of whether rights are meant to guarantee children's needs or their choices (Brennan 2002). There is a valid argument that it can and should happen the other way around: people need to be entitled and empowered to make claims on their rights to basic needs (provision). Because it is so easy to view orphans as especially vulnerable children, we have yet to see much action actually extending from such a rights-based premise in OVC programming.

From Protectionist Rights to Children's Citizenship

One way to reverse these alarming trends is to redouble efforts to use children's rights to promote orphans' empowerment—rather than their victimhood—through the development of more actionable legal protections for children. The new optional protocol is a good start. However, building more productive models for family, government, and NGO intervention on behalf of OVC lies not only in local and transnational discourses about orphans but also in rooting policy in a more nuanced understanding of AIDS-affected children's own experiences and their perceptions of their circumstances. Doing so may shift the discourse of humanitarian intervention toward augmenting children's agency, rather than ameliorating—and thereby sometimes deepening—their vulnerability.

To be effective, children's rights must also move from being a rhetorical, discursive device to an everyday, indigenous language that holds its own weight in social practice to build a culture of children's rights (Hanson and

Nieuwenhuys 2013). This shift may yield a greater sense of social justice for children, but it will rely on adults and adult institutions—whether local or global, rights-based or humanitarian-based—relinquishing their power over children and recognizing children's citizenship through more transformative models of assistance (Invernizzi and Milne 2005). Effecting such a drastic shift in attitude will not be easy, of course; in 2007, Dorothy Oulanyah, HIV specialist for OVC prevention in Uganda, admitted to me in an interview that UNICEF may have erred in its initial efforts to promote children's rights in Uganda:

> We started by telling people what children's rights were, and children quickly picked up on it . . . but then we got to a point where the children were running ahead of the parents and the rest of the community. Now, when you mention child rights in a community, they will say, "You are spoiling our children! Now we can't even discipline our children. We can't tell them what to do because you've come with this child rights message." So now we're trying to reverse that and say that children also have a right to parental guidance and put it in context so that it is not that children rule over you. But it's something so hard to reverse because we had such a big drive in the early 1990s, really pushing the issue.[4]

To overcome this backlash, not only must children's rights be reframed to emphasize participation in decision-making processes, but adults must come to see children's rights as beneficial to the entire community rather than as a tool that can either be manipulated or implemented at the expense of adults. Given that childhood is such a naturalized concept, however, that change will likely require a significant shift in both local and global understandings of children as rights bearers.

Citizenship is a more useful analytical framework for this task. As Allison James has pointed out, "adults' ideas about childhood limit children's agency and actions, thereby denying them status as citizens" (2011, 167). If children are seen as incomplete citizens-in-training, to be protected to foster the growth of complete (read: adult) citizens in the future, it is no wonder that rights-based approaches are not increasing children's empowerment: the cultural politics of childhood put forward in children's rights discourses tend to place children's citizenship in the future (James 2011). This sort of protectionism in the guise of rights is thus detrimental to children's citizenship. In the case of OVC in Africa, it affects their very survival. Yet, it should not be as hard to promote children's citizenship in Africa as international development discourse suggests: while "traditional culture" is often framed as the barrier to the fulfilment of children's rights, I have shown here how the protectionism of children's rights actually originates in Western concepts of the "precious child" (Zelizer 1985). In Africa, by contrast, children have long been comparatively more autonomous—while also more accountable to their communities (Whiting and Whiting 1975). However, due to the way rights tend to be individually conceptualized (i.e., granted to sovereign individuals rather than communities), OVC aid prescriptions can get applied in Africa as if the extended-family care systems are not already well established or are incapable of properly caring for children, thus undermining rather than bolstering their capacity to do so (Phiri and Tolfree 2005). So while many international rights organizations talk of the need to "sensitize" societies in the Global South to children's rights, perhaps the bigger issue is one of framing; for example, rooting children's rights discourse in indigenous knowledge so that it is not seen as alien or neocolonial but rather compatible with local understandings of children's social roles.[5] Thus, local constructions of childhood that acknowledge children's (deferential) contributions to their community have more potential to be harnessed by promoters of children's rights than does trying to impose Western constructions of the "precious but useless" child whose citizenship is placed in the future. The Uganda Child Rights NGO Network (UCRNN) has thus tried to localize children's rights by emphasizing children's responsibilities alongside their rights (Cheney 2007b, 60). As Nicola Taylor and Anne Smith point out, "The rights and duties of citizens are what make them full members of community. . . . Responsibilities for children are both activities that adults expect and are obliged to carry out, and activities that children find important to take care of in their own or other people's interest" (2009, 16). Contextualizing children's rights and responsibilities in this way makes them more compatible with local constructions of children as such contextualization supports recognition of children's contributions to family, community, and society—that is, their citizenship.

LACK OF CHILDREN'S PARTICIPATION
IN ORGANIZATIONAL CONTEXTS

Standards of participation in aid and development are applied differently in the case of children. Despite their stated goals to promote participation rights for children, many aid organizations gloss over this point in their own programming. When it comes to decision making within the organizations assisting children, participation efforts can be tokenistic at best.

An abundance of recent literature critiques the practice of child participation within aid programming as superficial and unsubstantive for the fulfillment of children's rights (Campbell 2008; de Waal and Argenti 2002; Evans

2007; Frankel 2007; Invernizzi and Milne 2002; Milne 2005). Aid organizations are often driven by international development agendas that use children's rights frameworks as a guide in designing participatory programming. While Save the Children argues that "participation transforms the power relations between children and adults, challenges authoritarian structures and supports children's capacity to influence families, communities and institutions" (Save the Children 2006, 33–34), these are the very reasons why aid organizations tend to resist children's participation, "because it disrupts adults' established working pattern and challenges existing norms" (A. West 2007, 126). If rights are to "hold powerful people and institutions accountable for their responsibilities to those with less power" (Save the Children 2006, 23), as if intergenerational power relations are a zero-sum game, they apparently are not necessarily going to shift the balance of power within children's rights organizations, instead maintaining the relationship of the weak relying on the powerful to grant them their rights. Even where rights discourses are not seen as foreign impositions, they can still fall short of participation goals when the protectionism that undergirds children's rights reinforces preexisting cultural presumptions—local, global, or organizational—of children's social incompetence. Children's participation is often limited in that it tends not to involve children at the decision-making level, reinforcing preexisting cultural attitudes that, while certainly not confined to my field site in Uganda, are prevalent there. Structural factors such as poverty and instability have made the fulfillment of children's rights particularly challenging in Africa, where children disproportionately suffer human rights violations (Ehlers and Frank 2008, 111). Further, cultural practices challenge government efforts to cultivate child participation. As John Okiror, manager of the Uganda OVC National Implementation Unit in 2009, pointed out to me, 'Uganda is a country which is rich culturally. We have so many different kinds of culture, and . . . most of these cultures, I think, treat children as people that are supposed just to take; they are not supposed to be listened to. They are supposed to take what an adult does."[6] Ugandan adults often think that children cannot contribute meaningfully to solving social problems or that children do not know what is good for them. Participation is thus the biggest challenge because of issues with both cultural and literal translation of the language of development (Cheney 2007b). Organizational cultivation of children's participation was hampered early on by efforts to educate children about their rights, as Oulanyah explained. Despite adjusting its strategies to stress parental guidance, UNICEF has found it difficult to reverse the backlash against children's rights.

Legal scholars Louise Ehlers and Cheryl Frank state that in Africa, "there is a lack of national policies that allow for the formal, ongoing participation of children. . . . Even amongst children's rights organizations, there have been few attempts to integrate the participation of children into the way in which these organizations do their business, and both national policy and general practices need to be addressed to accommodate this" (2008, 123–24). Though children have a right to participation, they are often excluded from aid and development programming, especially when considered vulnerable (Powell and Smith 2009). Given the complex yet concrete barriers to fulfillment of children's rights, creating opportunities for children to participate in policy making and NGO programming offers great promise for improving their overall situations. Recognizing this potential, in 2008, the Uganda Ministry of Gender, Labour, and Social Development worked together with UNICEF and the UCRNN to create a child participation guide for NGOs working in the country. But the booklet makes few references to the particular barriers in the local context (Uganda Ministry of Gender Labour and Social Development, Uganda Child Rights NGO Network, and UNICEF 2008), sticking instead to defining the broader principles of children's rights.

According to Ehlers and Frank, "The primary question that arises is how [participation efforts] should be evaluated in terms of their value for children in Africa?" (2008, 111). They enumerate four criteria for child participation: "that children involved understand the intentions of the project; that they know who made the decisions concerning their involvement, and why; that they have a meaningful role; and that they volunteer for the project after its nature has been made clear to them" (Ehlers and Frank 2008, 114). *Meaningful* is a highly subjective term in this context; I would further define *participation* as having a positive collective impact—however small—on the situations children face in the local context. Being able to affect policy by incorporating children's perspectives should be a primary outcome of any program's design goal. It must also work within the context of children's everyday realities rather than universals; otherwise, they may remain ineffective.

In Uganda, the OVC secretariat has tried to promote children's participation in its coordination of OVC programming by both government and NGO offices, but it tends to clash with cultural constructions of children that demand their silence and deference to adult opinion. Okiror told me that this was the biggest challenge because children do not tend to express their views, but who could blame them when most of their interaction with adult authority explicitly teaches them not to? Even the participation handbook that instructs organizations on how to involve children reproduces many prevalent stereotypes about children's inherently incompetent nature (Uganda Ministry of Gender, Labour, and Social Development, Uganda Child Rights NGO Network, and UNICEF 2008). This underlying reinforcement of stereotypes may quickly lead organizations to give up trying to respect, involve, and listen to children. If children are taught not to express their views, it will take time, patience, and the careful building of rapport with children to undo such socialization.

Even where people may be truly committed to child participation, it may emerge that staff within the same organization have conflicting ideas about what that actually means in practice (Naker 2007). This trend indicates that the deeper issues have to do with cultural presumptions (in Western and developing country contexts) about children as people who are dependent, seen but not heard, irrational, incompetent, and so on. The language of protection is then commonly used as an excuse for excluding children from participating in decision making that affects them, easily masking the fact that adults may not really want to do the work necessary to hear what children have to say. I do not wish to claim here that participation and protection are mutually exclusive. Indeed, guaranteeing children's citizenship also entails adults' protection of (particularly very young) children from harm for them to reach their full potential as citizens. On the contrary, they are mutually constitutive, as Powell and Smith nicely summarize:

> The nature of protection is a disputable concept, with overprotection seen as harmful. True protection of children requires all rights, including participation rights, to be respected. A distinction has been made between the inherent and the structural vulnerability of children. The inherent vulnerability of children, as a consequence of biological immaturity, emphasizes that researchers and significant adults in children's lives have an ethical responsibility to protect children. However, the structural vulnerability of children comes about as a consequence of, and subsequently serves to reinforce, social and political mechanisms that reduce children's power, fail to take their agency into account and disregard their rights. (Powell and Smith 2009, 138)

This dynamic demonstrates a conflict between children's right to be protected and their right to influence decisions that affect them. Accommodating children's participation may therefore involve adults learning to more effectively communicate with children, which will in turn require a greater attitude shift on the part of adults than of children. Thus, the challenge is not so much to convince children that they have something to say as to convince adults that children's opinions do indeed matter. Participation and citizenship go hand in hand: "The more children are treated and constructed as citizens, the more likely it is that they will actively participate in society," (Taylor and Smith 2006, 19), thereby claiming what Manfred Liebel (2012) calls "children's rights from below."

Recognition of OVC as citizens in Uganda may ironically have been set back by humanitarian interventions that reified orphans, set them apart from family contexts, and reinforced their "victim" status. Those who truly wish to protect children must first come to realize that participation itself may act as a means of protection by allowing children like Margaret access to opportunities and resources previously denied them (Powell and Smith 2009, 129). Further, encouraging participation builds citizenship skills in children that will strengthen fledgling democracies such as Uganda.

Policy makers and aid organizations would therefore do well to be more reflexive in their authoring and implementing of children's rights approaches, to overcome their own myopia in regard to advancing children's lived citizenship rather than deferring it to the future. Save the Children, for instance, mentions forms of discrimination and talks of "enabling children and young people from discriminated against groups to speak out and engage with decision makers" (Save the Children 2006, 32), going on to mention devices such as children's parliaments. It does not, however, go so far as to suggest children's representatives in actual state parliaments.[7] Is their assumption that governments are already watching out for children's interests, or that separate and unequal participation for children is sufficient for the fulfilment of their rights? The reality is that, from a rights perspective, children generally can be seen as a marginalized majority that is still discriminated against. The way these policies are constructed belies that simple fact, instead maintaining the status quo in which children may be protected but largely remain powerless to change their own circumstances by claiming their rights.

How should we deal with discrimination against children like Margaret; who are trying to seek services that will in fact protect them and provide for their own best interests in the absence or diminished capacity of adult caregivers? The achievement of lived rights and citizenship for children lies not only in emphasizing social and economic rights to alleviate the widespread poverty that drives global humanitarianism but also in recognizing children's capacity to act, legally and socially, on their own behalf to secure the resources necessary for survival. Until the promise of children's rights can be used to help advance children's lived citizenship, however, orphans like Margaret will continue to embrace their vulnerabilities to seek care, wherever and from whomever it is available. While some orphans will gain certain entitlements this way, this practice will ultimately uphold their collective marginalization, thereby denying their participation rights.

These strategies can be seen in themselves as agentive acts on the part of the vulnerable: on an up-country trip with UWESO staff members in 2009 to visit their projects and talk with some of their clients, I spent the afternoon with some children whose families benefited from UWESO income-generating programs. They were shy at first, but when we starting kicking around a soccer ball, they loosened up and started joking with one another, trying out their English on me. They seemed to think they were speaking my language in more ways than one: one child said to another, "You are an orphan. You need special care!" They laughed as they enumerated their own vulnerabilities, all the while keeping the ball moving.

Getting Children's Perspectives: A Child- and Youth-Centered Participatory Approach

As in organizational settings, children are rarely involved in research, except as objects. If we as researchers are to avoid the same pitfalls of participation, we need to remedy that lack of involvement by adopting more inclusive methodologies in our research with young people. Children have long been objects of anthropological analysis—through studies of child rearing, for example—but research on children's own experiences of social processes is a rather recent phenomenon (Hirschfeld 2002). While conducting previous research with children in Uganda in 2000–2001, I therefore pursued what I have called *child-centered ethnography* (Cheney 2007b): attention to the ways children act, not just as objects of socialization but as social agents and cultural producers (James, Jenks, and Prout 1998), following the pioneering work of childhood studies, which has since flourished into a burgeoning field in its own right. Despite the attention scholars have given to children's agency, there is still considerable resistance to more participatory methods wherein children could exercise that agency.

In this chapter, I argue that ethnographic research, the hallmark methodology of anthropology, is particularly appropriate to the task not only of capturing the lived experiences of children as a distinct social group but also of increasing both children's participation and children's citizenship—especially when it models children's participation in its own research design. Despite the challenges of incorporating children and youth participation into research design itself, I felt it important for this project in order to tell a different story about AIDS orphanhood from the points of view of young people. While this method was not without its challenges, the benefits of involving children as ethnographers that I discuss in this chapter far outweighed any drawbacks. These benefits included establishing greater rapport to challenge assumptions about children's limited competencies. As I hope to show in this discussion of the research methodology I employed in this project, participatory ethnographic research with children is essential to the task of better understanding children's everyday situations in any given social context.

I first contextualize the project in broader discussions about child participation in research. I then discuss the research design and its challenges, limitations, and benefits.

Locating Children's Participation

Social researchers have written a number of books and articles addressing the issue of research with children (Alderson and Morrow 2011; Christensen and James 2000; Hirschfeld 2002; James 2007). While social scientists have shifted a more significant gaze toward children's lives, Pia Christensen and Alan Prout have also acknowledged that, at least within academic research, "the perspective of 'children as social actors' has created a field with new ethical dilemmas and responsibilities for researchers within the social study of childhood" (2002, 477). We cannot therefore critique organizational practices for their lack of children's participation without also interrogating the correlative absence of children in social research.

As an engaged anthropologist in childhood and international development studies, I too often focus in my presentations on what is *not* working for children in Africa; how, for example, institutions both local and global fail to create meaningful structural changes to improve the lives of children, or even avenues of participation for them, due to a protectionist—rather than empowering—interpretation of children's rights (Cheney 2014a). I am often asked, "Then what would real participation look like?" This is indeed the question: though scholars and practitioners alike will claim—rightly or not—that participation is a pillar of the United Nations Convention on the Rights of the Child (CRC), we do not always practice what we preach: children were not involved in the drafting or implementation of the CRC (Boyden 1997, 222). And though there are valid arguments that children are not always capable of making policy, Judith Ennew (2002) noted that the CRC makes no distinction between the competencies of seventeen-month-old and seventeen-year-old children. In any case, there is little agreement about what constitutes meaningful child participation; where some may find one model sufficiently participatory as long as it, say, involves young people in some consultative way, others criticize it as tokenist or even exploitative (Groundwater-Smith, Dockett, and Bottrell 2015, 32–33).

As mentioned in chapter 3, the tension between protectionist and par-

ticipatory or empowering approaches with children carries over into organizational contexts. While many organizations, governmental and nongovernmental, are working hard to promote children's rights in Uganda, they
often find it counterintuitive to work with children on even a semiequal level,
opting instead to implement children's rights according to the "best interest
principle," which posits that the fulfillment of children's rights must still lie
in the hands of adults who know what is best for children. While this approach does indeed often serve to protect children, it can also work to their
disadvantage. Predominant ideas about childhood and intergenerational relationships also come to bear on children's possibilities for participation in
decisions that affect them. However, John Okiror, manager of the Uganda
OVC (orphans and vulnerable children) National Implementation Unit in
2009, told me that implementing participatory practices is also a matter of
convincing children that they have something to contribute. This revelation
should come as no surprise, since adults are well aware that social norms and
constructions of childhood have conditioned children *not* to voice their opinions. This conditioning most certainly will not be undone by suddenly admit-
ting children into the boardroom. Even in my research with children, I often
find that it takes considerable time for me to build rapport, mainly because
children are prepared to listen to me rather than having me listen to them.
They are often initially baffled by my wanting to learn from them and need
encouragement—even permission—to talk freely. At the same time, though,
practitioners, policy makers, and researchers are confronted with yielding
their authority to younger people, which is also counterintuitive to the adult
constructions of intergenerational relations in which they are ensconced.
Andy West of Save the Children China suggests, "A first step toward overcoming resistance to participation is to understand local social constructions
of childhood and how they might impact participatory work. . . . Adult practitioners . . . must actually engage with children in order to expand their pre-
conceived constructions of childhood" (A. West 2007, 131). This sounds like
an anthropological enterprise, which drives home how aid and development
organizations might benefit from involving more anthropologists in their research: this insight is obvious to them. Participatory research methods admittedly lend themselves better to interpretive research endeavors than positivist
ones, hence child participation and anthropological or ethnographic research
are compatible and can be mutually constitutive. Ethnographic research is
also good at revealing the incongruities of cultural intersections, particularly
between universalized ideals, the institutions that operationalize them, and
local communities. In the case of a concept such as *childhood*, such incongru-
ity has social justice implications for children as a social group—and because

participatory methods also lend themselves well to research projects with a social justice component, they seemed the natural choice while planning this study. In any case, researchers cannot well critique various social institutions for excluding children from meaningful participation and then do the same. But this was not the only reason I opted for this approach: it has merits in its own right, including authenticity of the findings.

Participatory Research Design: Creating Spaces for Young People's Participation

In this research project, I wanted to address the power dynamics of research, not only between adults and children in development but within knowledge production *about* children *by* adults, as well as about Africa by the West. I also wanted to know young people's perspectives on orphanhood. I thus developed my research design with these epistemological questions in mind. I wanted to conduct this study by better incorporating children's concerns in ways that emphasized children's participation not just as respondents but as people who help shape the research design, so that young researchers could contribute to the amelioration of their own and others' difficult circumstances (Ehlers and Frank 2008, 116). I also tried to incorporate these ethical considerations into the research design.

When I conducted previous research with children in Uganda, I became keenly aware of the rising number of orphans, mainly as a result of the AIDS epidemic. When I returned to Uganda in the summer of 2007 to start this project on AIDS orphanhood, I was heavily invested in finding ways to continue to work with the children and families with which I had built relationships on past visits to Uganda—not only to draw on my existing resources but also to help people I knew network with one another in ways that would continue to benefit them in their personal, educational, and career goals. I also wanted to go beyond lip service about "giving voice" to children. Allison James, one of the scholars credited with initiating a new paradigm for childhood studies in the late 1980s and early 1990s, thinks that the 1980s "writing culture" debates in anthropology have contemporary salience for child researchers. In 2007, she posited that "current rhetoric about 'giving voice to children' . . . poses a threat to the future of childhood research because it masks a number of important conceptual and epistemological problems." These problems include "questions of representation, issues of authenticity, the diversity of children's experiences, and children's participation in research" (James 2007, 261). In trying to respond to such concerns, I wanted my research to be not only participatory but also collaborative and decolonizing.

Collaborative Research with Young People

Working in a team can be a challenge for an ethnographer: anthropologists typically claim to work alone, or only marginally with local people, when the truth is that every research participant, every friend and cultural guide, is a collaborator in building our cultural interpretations. I decided to list these people among my best assets for the project by inviting former child research participants and community stakeholders to be involved in shaping the research design to better reflect their concerns about orphanhood. Because their own lives have been affected by HIV/AIDS and orphanhood, it also provides a longitudinal perspective on the experience.

Fieldwork for this volume was conducted mainly from 2007 to 2009, during which time youth research assistants (RAs) did the primary data collection. Research coordinator Faridah Ddamulira and I also made follow-up visits together to the study community between 2011 and 2015. The study was conducted in a periurban area of Kampala with thirty-nine children and their families, along with key informant interviews with representatives of government and nongovernmental organization (NGO) offices. I first approached a community school to which I had initially been introduced in 1993 and with which my family and I had been associated since. I knew that many families affected by HIV/AIDS lived in the area and that the school catered to orphans and destitute children. I worked with Faridah, the niece of the friend who had introduced me to the school. Faridah had grown up in the community and held a social sciences degree from Makerere University.

PRELIMINARY RESEARCH

Faridah and I began by identifying participants at the school. Not wanting to explicitly single out children whose parents had died, we had children draw pictures of their homes and the people who lived there. Through interviews with the children about their drawings, we learned of the children's general circumstances at their homes, and thus we were able to identify orphans and other vulnerable children without having to ask them directly whether they were orphans. This process also gave us a chance to see how the children would interact with us, in groups and individually. We organized those children into five focus groups, roughly one for each class from kindergarten through third grade, and met with them several times per week during free periods at school. This regular interaction allowed us to build profiles of each child, with basic information on their home and family circumstances (see appendix). We also contacted households with children who were out of school so as to compare.

I wanted to maintain relationships with previous informants as well. The children featured in my book *Pillars of the Nation* (Cheney 2007b) had since grown up; by 2007, they were all in their late teens to early twenties and were nearing completion of their secondary school studies. I had been in touch with some of them and had helped them with their schooling; others I had lost touch with and was able to relocate only when I returned (I provide updates on these children in chapter 5). Several of them were orphaned themselves, which had jeopardized their ability to complete education and get job training skills. If I trained them as youth research assistants, I reasoned, they would bring their direct experience of orphanhood to the project as well as superior cultural and linguistic knowledge to my own. Given that they were younger than me—and thus closer in age to our current study participants—this research design would yield more genuine data and allow young people, both the child participants and the older youth research assistants, to have greater overall input into the research process. Finally, the design also made pragmatic sense, since I would only be able to visit to conduct research on my holidays from teaching, I could set up the research team to conduct the research such that they could continue while I could not be there.

I thus decided I would try to involve the young people who were described in *Pillars of the Nation* (Cheney 2007b)—under the pseudonyms James, Jill, Malik, Michael, and Sumayiya—as research assistants, providing compensation for transportation and supply costs and incentive through financial assistance for school.

Once I had decided on this approach and all five of the young people I contacted had accepted, I was still daunted by the task of figuring out how to teach them how to do social research—until I remembered my old friends Martin Geria and Simon Opolot of the African Training, Research, and Innovation Network (A-TRAIN). I had known these two friends since my first visit to Uganda in 1993. They had formed A-TRAIN in the early years of the twenty-first century to, as they wrote in their promotional material, "foster recovery, growth and development in Africa through training, research, innovation and networking in the creation, acquisition, adaptation and application of knowledge that has become a key factor in the stimulation and promotion of growth and development." I knew they had already designed training programs for participatory action research in refugee communities, so I approached them about conducting a workshop with my potential youth research assistants to get them acquainted with social research principles and methods. My A-TRAIN friends decided they could conduct a two-day work-shop that would get the youth RAs started, and then we could have occasional follow-up workshops that would allow the youth RAs to learn by doing as we came together to address issues, discuss findings, and decide on new direc-tions for the research design. In the meantime, Faridah would help the youth RAs with logistical and methodological support.

THE FIRST YOUTH RESEARCH ASSISTANT WORKSHOP

When the day came for the youth RA workshop at the end of my summer stay in 2007, I was really anxious: could we pull it off? Could we get buy-in from all the stakeholders we had involved, from children to guardians to youth RAs? We got started, and as soon as Simon launched into the first session, I had no further doubts; he was expert at explaining things in a clear and concise man-ner that engaged the young people from the start (fig. 3). The information was also well laid out so that the participants picked it up quickly. If they were still

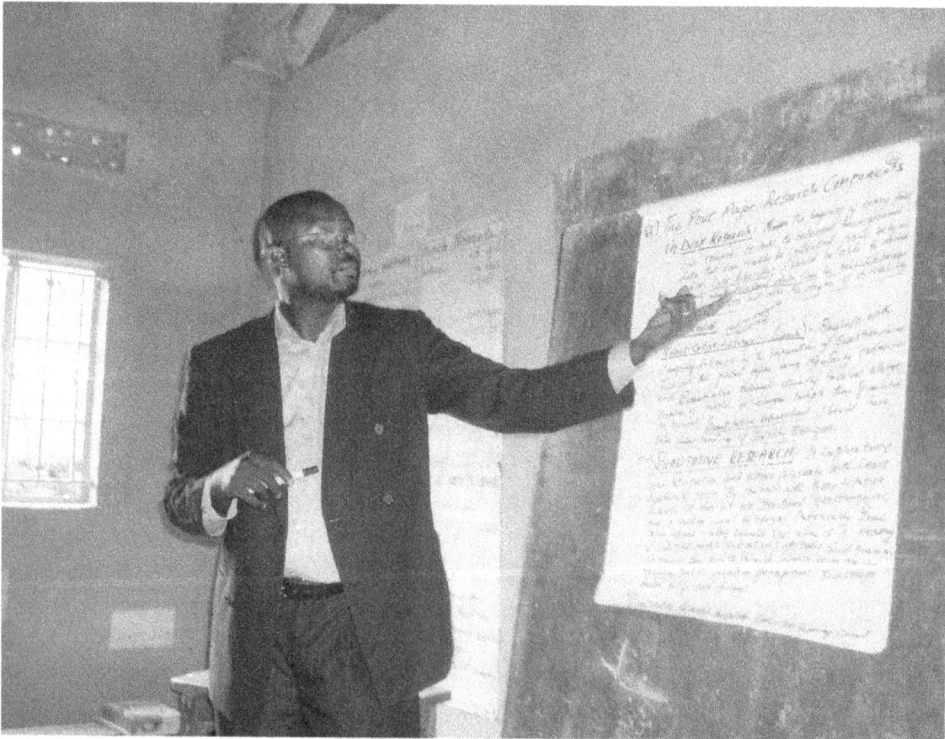

FIGURE 3. Simon Opolot of the African Training, Research, and Innovation Network (A-TRAIN) pre-sents information at the first youth research assistant workshop in July 2007.

reserved when Martin took over the next session, he cleared the air with his humor and some entertaining icebreakers.

We covered such methods as participant observation, focus group discussions, and interviewing, allowing the youth RAs to practice on us and one another. When we talked about the ethics of working with a vulnerable population of children, I was able to remind the youth RAs how intimidated they might have felt when they talked to me initially back in 2000. I told them how we chose the study participants without making them feel as though they were singled out for being orphans, and Sumayiya described how awful it felt when that had happened to her as a child. She even volunteered that she had hidden her orphanhood by calling her aunt and uncle Mom and Dad so that other children would not know and treat her differently—a fact she had previously concealed even in front of the other youth RAs who had been her schoolmates when she was younger. Jill and Michael also responded well to questions, and James really took to the recording equipment—a real gadget guy. They were also observant of our warnings that they keep children's information confidential (especially HIV status—see chapter 6) and be mindful of guardians' and other gatekeepers' concerns.

In consultation with Faridah, I had assigned each youth RA one in-school focus group and one out-of-school household (see the appendix for a complete list). On the second day, I distributed the RAs' Focus Group Profiles we had developed after the initial picture-drawing activity and interview about the picture. Faridah and I gave them some pointers for interacting with individual children. We warned that the children might be reserved at first—as they were with us—but that they would likely loosen up before long. The goal at this point was just to let the children get used to the youth RAs and gain a little familiarity with them. The youth RAs looked intimidated, so I reminded them that the thought of working with them when they were young was also initially intimidating to me. They just had to remember to relate to the children on their own terms, what Christensen and Prout have referred to as "ethical symmetry," that is, "that the researcher takes as his or her starting point the view that the ethical relationship between researcher and informant is the same whether he or she conducts research with adults or with children ... [and that] any difference between carrying out research with children or with adults should be allowed to arise from this starting point, according to the concrete situation of children, rather than being assumed in advance" (Christensen and Prout 2002, 482).

We went into the classroom to meet the thirty-nine focus group children, who had all come dressed in their Sunday best. Wide-eyed, they stared at us. The headmistress of the school, here called by the pseudonym Josephine, had told them that we had brought them new teachers because she thought that would make it easier for the children to relate to the new researchers. But to break down the sense of us as authority figures, we preferred to approach them as friends. Still, they stood and greeted us, and Josephine introduced us by testing them on my and Faridah's names. They had no problem with that. She turned to Martin and Simon and asked the children how we should regard them: as fathers, uncles, or *jaajas* (grandfathers)? Definitely *jaajas*, the children decided after sizing them up for a moment. We all laughed, but Martin and Simon went along willingly with what the children wanted.

Each of the youth RAs introduced themselves, ad-libbing here and there to put the children at ease by being open, friendly, and easy to get to know. We sent each youth RA with his or her focus group to separate classrooms, and they all went to work, playing and singing and generally doing things that the children really enjoyed. As I walked around and saw how the youth RAs were adjusting to fit the children's needs, I knew with absolute certainty that we had pulled it off; this project would go forward. The children connected almost instantly with their new youth RAs as friends and even brothers and sisters. Martin surmised that it was because Faridah and I had primed the children well to receive new friends, but I think the youth RAs also did a great job of making them feel comfortable. For example, Malik was assigned to a focus group comprised solely of second-grade children from the home of a woman known in the community as Jaaja (Grandma) Rose, a guardian of fourteen children at the time. Malik asked them where they lived, and they pointed toward their house just down the hill from the school. "Right over there!" they all chimed in.

"And who do you live with?" he asked. They all clammed up, perhaps anticipating a little of the discrimination that orphans living in grandparents' and other extended families' homes sometimes experience.

"We live with our *jaaja*," one of them finally volunteered hesitantly.

"Oh, really? I was raised by my *jaaja,* too." Malik replied. This revelation caused them to do a double take, and they quickly sized Malik up. It looked to them like he had done all right, and that reassured them. The kids from Jaaja Rose's house began to draw their home and tell Malik all about their family (fig. 4). Before long, Shekinah was hanging off Malik's leg and Travis, who had been quite reserved up until then, was jumping into even my arms.

Even James quickly figured out how to appeal to his group of five-year-old kindergarteners by singing and playing games, and a lot of them shared information with the children, who responded by answering questions. Sumayiya took to little Raj in her second-grade group and observed that despite his small size, he dominated the group with his strong personality. Jill connected

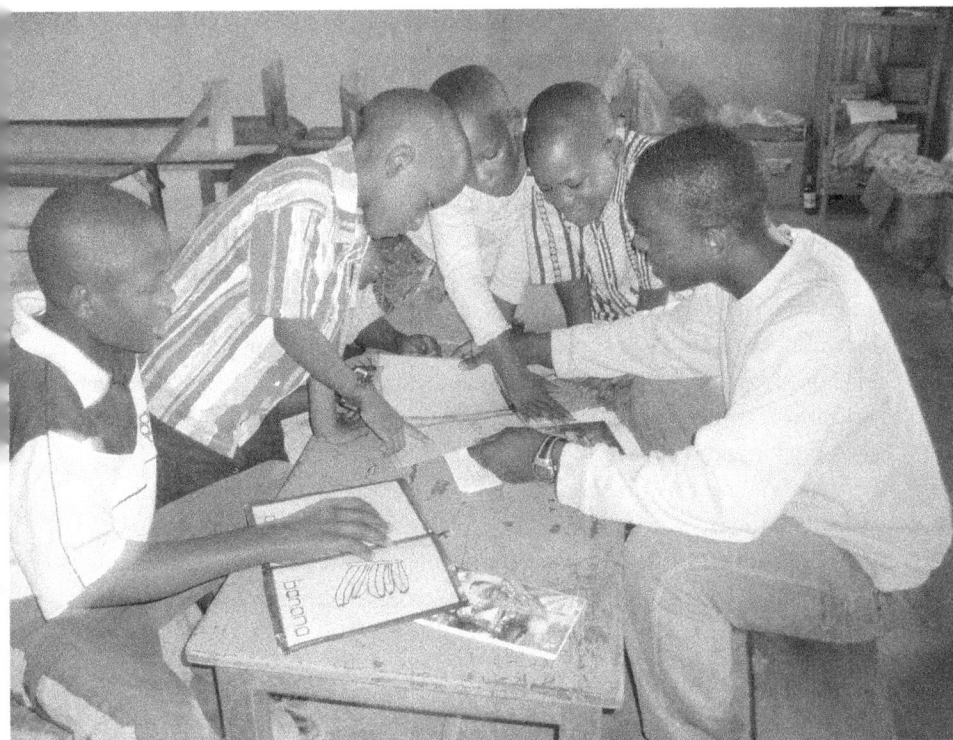

FIGURE 4. Youth research assistant Malik (*right*) gets acquainted with the children in his focus group in July 2007.

with her third-grade girls by playing netball. Even the usually sullen second-grade boys Wasswa and Carter in Malik's group were all smiles.

The children had warmed to Faridah and me by the time we conducted the workshop, but with the youth RAs, they were downright affectionate. I could see it all in motion now: how this research design would not only produce more intimate knowledge of these children's lives but also connect people in the research community with one another in meaningful ways that would radiate out from the project itself. When we came back together to reflect a bit before lunch, the youth RAs were all fired up. They noted how easy it was when they related to children on their own terms and let them be themselves. And they were also impressed with how easy it was for the children to share information with them when they put the children at ease. They were excited to get back to the children to eat lunch with them, so they gathered up their teams behind them and lined up to get some of Jaaja Rose's delicious beans, rice, and cabbage.

Simon was also pleased to realize that this project could have lasting effects in that the youth RAs we were talking with that day could even choose social research as a career path or perhaps go on to work for other projects meant to improve service delivery to vulnerable children. Even head teacher Josephine, who participated in the workshop, realized that she had been doing community-based research for a long time—whenever she interacted with the children and their families in ways that benefited the children. I could also see that, beyond my interests in conducting research being served, A-TRAIN had provided the youth RAs with marketable skills that would also help them as they moved from school into the job market; it networked members of the research team with new people in their community, yielding possible future collaborations; youth RAs and study participants created instant mentoring bonds. In fact, we were quickly hearing questions from the children about when they would see their "big brothers and big sisters" again.

At the end of the workshop, we awarded certificates of completion to the youth RAs (fig. 5). Certificates of completion of trainings are important résumé builders in Uganda, and many people carry a portfolio of such certificates to job interviews. We took a few pictures before dispersing slowly. It

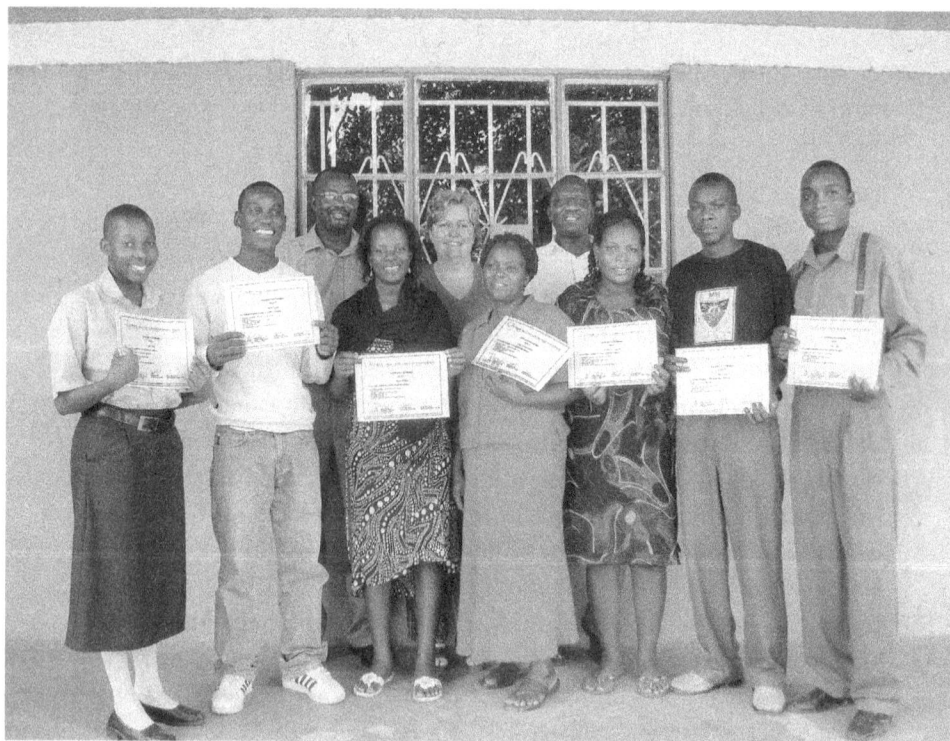

FIGURE 5. Youth research assistants receive certificates of completion of initial training in July 2007.

had been such a successful workshop, though, that no one seemed to want to go home.

DATA COLLECTION

The youth RAs were asked to make regular visits (at least once a month) to each of the children in their focus groups, at school and at home, for a period of two years. Using a set of guiding questions about orphans' circumstances and survival strategies, the youth RAs engaged with the children through the various methods they had learned. They each kept a journal of field notes. They were in regular contact with Faridah, who assisted whenever they ran into trouble or had immediate questions, and Faridah reported back to me on how the youth RAs and the children they visited were doing. Whenever I could return, we held workshops, and each youth RA would provide updates on each of the children in their focus groups (fig. 6).

To help maintain a sense of young people's authority in the research design, I used the data chain model of Pryor and Ampiah (2004). In a data chain, collected data act as a stimulus for dialogue to interpret the data and produce and verify findings. We could generate new data from the research teams' recognition of patterns among the children with whom they worked. We could then form narratives and generate new questions and goals for the next phase of the research. For example, if we found a phenomenon to be common among the children (the "what"), we could then plan to investigate the phenomenon to get a deeper understanding of the "how" and the "why." We would build our data chain over the course of six total youth RA workshops in the two years we conducted the main study. We developed data chains by coming together every four to six months to share findings made by individual youth RAs and then looking for commonalities among their reports. I thus relinquished much of my authority as the principal investigator to privilege the children's and youth RAs' knowledge as the "experts" on their own lives. I would often ask questions about whether a certain interpretation I was developing from their data was accurate, and this inquiry would lead us into prolonged and nuanced discussions about observed social phenomena concerning orphans, social actions, and their meanings. We would collectively answer some questions but invariably yield new ones—which translated into the next research task for the youth RAs.

Many of the research team's conversations centered on methodological concerns, so the workshops also became opportunities to continue to strengthen their research skills. It emerged that sometimes youth RAs would be unnecessarily rigid or data driven in their interactions with the children.

I encouraged the youth RAs to draw on their experiences of having been my research participants when they were younger and ponder these interactions: What stall tactics did they employ if they didn't feel like chatting with me on any given day? How did I react to them at the time? What responses to their feelings would they have appreciated? This line of questioning helped them understand how the children they were working with might perceive them and to adjust their research strategies to better honor the children's needs and wishes while still accomplishing the data collection task at hand.

The youth RA workshops were often the most constructive and informative conversations we had while conducting this research. Usually starting with a recap of the previous session, not only were they useful in research de-

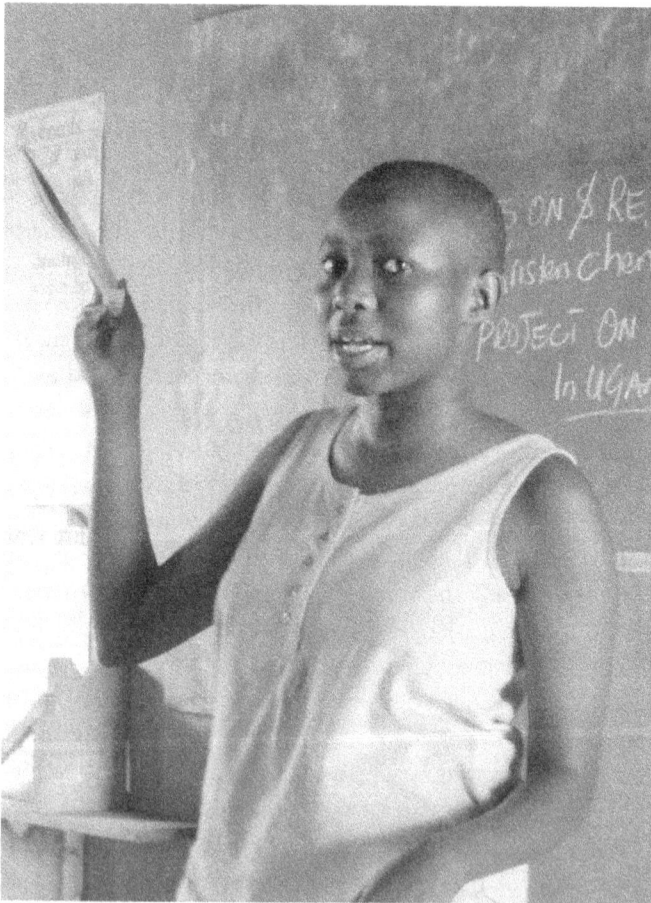

FIGURE 6. Youth research assistant Jill reports on the children in her focus group at first follow-up workshop, December 2007.

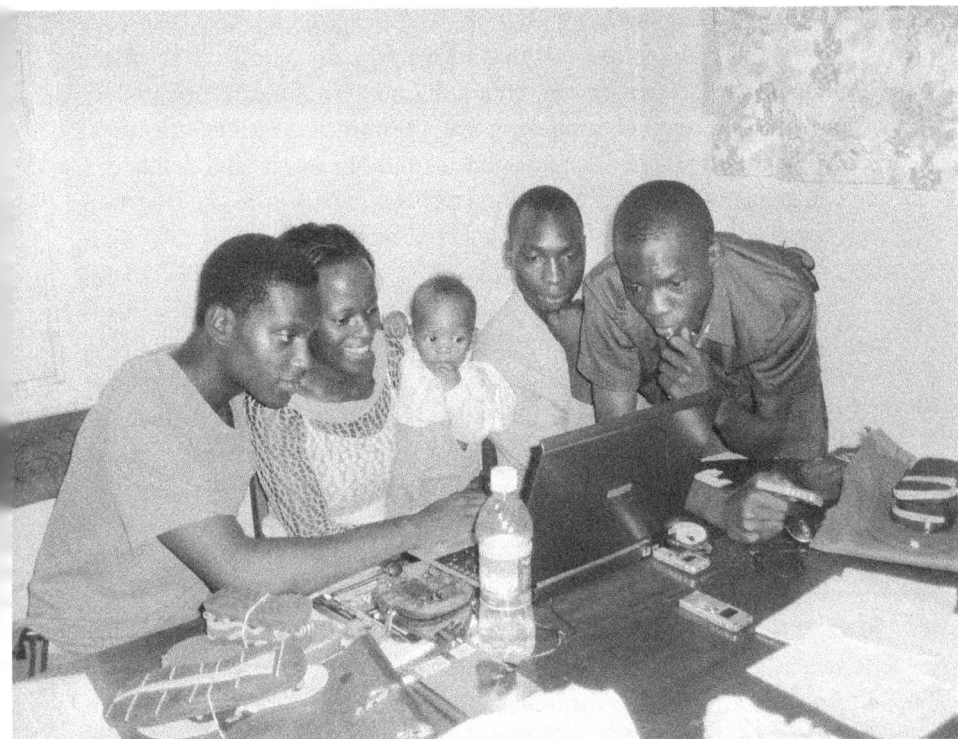

FIGURE 7. Youth research assistants go over data together at a workshop in 2008.

sign, but they also gave the youth RAs a chance to show how they were growing in skills and knowledge about the predicaments of children in their focus groups—and by extension, where appropriate, about orphans in general. It was also an opportunity for them to raise questions in an open forum so that we could all troubleshoot together about the challenges of fieldwork (fig. 7).

Decolonizing Research with African Children

> Research itself has been described as a colonizing construct . . . summarized as "they came, they saw, they named, they claimed."
>
> LINDA TUHIWAI SMITH, quoted in Mutua and Swadener 2004

Aside from being a question of rights and participation, participatory research with young people is a means of decolonizing the research process— and this makes it a matter of social justice. Research in Africa poses a number of ethical issues with which anthropologists continually struggle: Are we ever able to escape our disciplinary beginnings in the colonial enterprise? Are we still "claiming by naming"? Are we taking knowledge production away from local people by virtue of the fact that we are typically outsiders? These are valid questions that must be answered in the context of the history and development of Africanist anthropology. Despite the incredible influence of Africa on the development of the discipline of anthropology (Bates, Mudimbe, and O'Barr 1993; Schumaker 2001) and vice versa (Falk Moore 1994), African societies still understandably have trouble embracing anthropological knowledge. Because anthropology's beginnings were intertwined with colonial enterprises, there remains a dearth of native anthropologists in Africa, perhaps more than on any other continent. Only a handful of African universities to this day have their own anthropology departments, absorbing a few anthropologists into sociology departments instead (Ntarangwi, Mills, and Babiker 2006, 27–28). Those African anthropologists who do gain academic positions in university departments find research funding hard to come by unless, like many of their colleagues, they can secure contracts for applied work within development and aid organizations. So while it may not be ideal that Western anthropologists continue to produce the bulk of ethnographic texts on Africa, this situation has partly been due not only to a lack of resources but also to a lack of will on the part of African institutions to develop their own anthropological programs—at least to the extent that, say, Latin American universities have done.

Until that happens, we're it. It may not be possible for Western, Africanist anthropologists like me to completely overcome the legacies of colonialism and their collusion in anthropology's development, but I do not think that that renders the work of Western anthropologists working in former colonies itself colonizing or irrelevant. In their book *African Anthropologies: History, Critique, and Practice*, Mwenda Ntarangwi, David Mills, and Mustafa Babiker state, "Whilst one may wish to dismiss anthropology as an intimate part of colonial knowledge structure, one also has to acknowledge the interstitial space that the discipline offered to those of a critical bent, both in nurturing an anti-colonial consciousness and in inviting the first steps in Africanising the discipline" (2006, 19). It may not be transformational to do anthropological fieldwork in and of itself, but many Western anthropologists have proven that they *can* engage in critical work aimed at changing colonizing structures in African societies.

To me, decolonizing research means acknowledging the hegemonic practices involved in research dominated by Western social scientists—whether working with adults or children—and doing whatever possible to avoid or minimize any negative impact. Doing so involves interrogating privilege and the "myths of meritocracy" (one's own and those of one's informants) while strengthening local alliances, studying the languages and cultures to the degree possible, and developing the ability to code-switch and understand indigenous "ways of knowing" and communicating; providing equitable compensation for collaborators; making findings available in relevant ways to local shareholders; and participating in the ongoing development of scholarship in nonmissionary ways (Mutua and Swadener 2004). For me, this means actually utilizing the privilege I have as an educated white American to do work that has transformative potential for the population I study, mainly African children. It is in that spirit that I designed and conducted this research.

I do not believe it is ultimately me who decides whether I have achieved the goal of decolonization of the research; that is really for my informants and collaborators to decide. Declaring my research design colonization-free could in itself be labeled a colonizing move. As Harry West has noted about his own fieldwork, "Whereas postmodern critics might suggest that my interpretative vision of the Muedan life-world has 'silenced' Muedans themselves, I dare say the Muedans with whom I worked expected me—like anyone else—to speak assertively and authoritatively, articulating as convincingly as I was able my vision of the world we shared" (2007, 84). My collaborators have developed similar expectations of me over the years. I like to think of what I do in my research as holding up a mirror to help the people I work with see their own society more clearly—but I must acknowledge that that mirror does not capture everything in its purview, especially at the periphery. Ultimately, anthropology is an imperfect science, though as such it is one that has constantly struggled to improve itself, especially since the "crisis of representation" of the 1980s (Clifford and Marcus 1986). Still, I got into anthropology because I had a keen sense of social justice that needed satisfying, and I thought anthropology could make a difference in an increasingly interconnected if imperfect world. And so I continue to try—by sharing my interests, funding, and findings with local stakeholders, including young people. My African colleagues and students have appreciated these decolonizing efforts, and feedback from the youth RAs in our final workshop indicated that they not only learned more than they expected to about the plight of orphans around them, but they also learned a lot about themselves, both in terms of their own childhoods and in terms of their capabilities as youth researchers—a benefit that has had a lasting effect.

Challenges to Participatory Research with Children

Participatory research with young people was not without its challenges, however; the youth RA workshops became occasions for RAs to note some challenges with their research, and we discussed how to address them. Their obstacles were mainly environmental: it was too loud and disruptive to conduct interviews at school and even at the children's homes; guardians wanted to listen in, thereby inhibiting the responses of the children; children's friends were also disruptive; the timing of school holidays made it difficult to schedule visits; the children could get tired of answering the same questions repeatedly. These were in fact some of the same challenges I had encountered when doing research with the youth RAs themselves when they were younger participants in my previous study. For example, Jill said that one time she went to visit Pearl, one of the girls in her focus group, and her guardian said Pearl was in the field riding her bicycle, so they sent someone to fetch her. Jill waited an hour before Pearl came to the house, and Jill got the impression that Pearl was resentful that she was called from playing to sit down and do an interview. She was therefore rather uncooperative on that day. I recommended that, according to a Malawian proverb I had picked up while in Peace Corps, "if you find your friends roasting eyes, you should join them." In other words, I suggested that instead of pulling the children away from their usual activities, perhaps the youth RAs should consider joining them in those activities. I reminded them of when they were young and I would join them in schoolyard games. They had assumed that they needed to secure a recorded, sit-down interview, but I assured them that it would be all right if they went to the field with the children, observed, and wrote those observations later in their field notes. I suggested that all youth RAs go to the children instead of expecting the children to come to them, thus seizing the opportunity to conduct more participant observation. I urged the youth RAs to exercise patience; they might even learn a little more about the children in the process. At the same time, several youth RAs were complaining that guardians would hover over them when they visited children at home, concerned that they were being discussed; by going to where the children were, the youth RAs would be able to work better with the children on their own terms while also evading the guardians' surveillance.

James in particular met some emotional challenges when two children in his focus group, both from the same family, died of AIDS-related illnesses within several weeks of each other. Though he did not yet know them well, it really saddened him to see the way their grandmother suffered afterward. But, he noted, it also made him more empathetic with the children. "In fact," he noted, "I really didn't pay much attention to or even like children much before doing this project," but now he is much more interested in children's welfare in general. Faridah too was affected by the children's deaths, but through participating in the research, she said she had gained more sensitivity to people's problems; it had given her insight into the conditions of her community and made her more motivated to help.

For me, coordination of the research team was a difficult transition. Having always done my fieldwork solo, I had to adapt from being a hands-on field researcher to taking a more supervisory role. Until I was able to secure external funding that allowed me to obtain course release from my institution to stay for longer than six weeks at a time, I often felt relegated to the position of logistical officer—and bank: because the project involved sending six other people to the field on a regular basis, it was expensive. For the first year and a half, the vast majority of funds came out of my own pocket, as did the school fees I offered my youth RAs as compensation for their assistance. And yet the quality of observation and data I received from the youth RAs tended to vary. There were numerous reasons for this: some youth RAs just showed more motivation or propensity for doing fieldwork; some did good fieldwork but did not keep detailed field notes. In those instances, it was helpful to work with the youths' individual talents. For instance, Malik, a musician, did not feel adept at writing field notes, especially in English. But he was fascinated with the digital recorders. So I encouraged him to record his field notes orally and had them transcribed. James was similarly keen to use the video camera, so I had him work with it more extensively. Some of the youth RAs had family issues or illnesses that prevented them from conducting research as often as promised. The collaborative nature of the work drove research forward but at the same time made compilation of data, and thus its analysis, considerably slower—albeit more rewarding.

GATEKEEPERS AND ACCESS

I often find that the main challenges of working with children have less to do with children themselves than with their adult interlocutors. Adults—especially gatekeepers such as parents, guardians, and teachers—are often understandably protective (as their roles require). But they can also be uncomfortable with researchers' motivations for talking to the children in their care. Indeed, they are usually puzzled by researchers' actions: why don't we just talk to them, the guardians, about their children's needs? They can tell us everything we want to know! Sometimes guardians were worried that children in their care might report information to the youth RAs that might make them "look bad." Even though the youth RAs were "native" researchers who might share similar ideas about child rearing, guardians knew that the information might be shared with a wider audience and so wished to control the researchers' interactions with children as much as possible. To counter this tendency, I held several meetings with guardians of children during the initial phase of the study to temper expectations by stating explicitly what this study would—and would not—do for them and their children. While this tactic admittedly met with only partial success (as some only heard what they wanted to hear), it was important to make this attempt to secure their support for the project.

Just as organizations and researchers resist children's engagement because it can disrupt the normative ways of doing things (A. West 2007, 126), other adult interlocutors can resist children's participation in research to protect their own interests. Though all guardians gave their consent for us to work with their children, it soon became apparent that some did so only in the belief that they might secure some material or financial benefit.

One answer to this concern is to design research around the children's concerns themselves by, for instance, incorporating play into research or allowing children to identify their own needs and concerns. Flexibility must be built in from the beginning. Luckily, ethnographic projects tend to be flexible by their exploratory nature—the "deep hanging out" of participant observation, to borrow from Clifford Geertz (1998). This flexibility becomes even more advantageous when working with children, whose perspectives are routinely undervalued, especially in certain cultural contexts where children themselves often internalize predominant adult attitudes that children lack competence or cannot possibly be bearers of knowledge—even about childhood. Meeting and spending time with children in multiple spaces outside adult surveillance, such as joining children in play, helps overcome those obstacles.[1]

TEMPERING COMMUNITY EXPECTATIONS

Ethical considerations were numerous (and are discussed in more detail in subsequent chapters), but the issue of most conversation among the youth RAs was the expectations of the community. Community members were more likely to accept me if they thought I was an aid worker because they anticipated material compensation for their family's participation in the study. Designing research on orphans to include young Ugandan research assistants had the added advantage of removing me from regular contact with the families of the children and thus from their expectations. This distancing might seem like a *dis*advantage—and in some ways it certainly was—but it must be placed in the context of the community's increasing interactions with the aid industry: given the high expectations the community held of white foreigners (*azungu*) who come taking an interest in orphans, my absence served to temper those expectations. They did not completely disappear, however: by becoming research assistants, the youth RAs inadvertently became proxies for me as principal investigator, as well as outsiders within; the caregivers perceived them as having an elevated status—but one they could still manipulate by virtue of being elders dealing with young people, whom they expected to be subservient to them. Though I had tried to be as clear as possible from the beginning about the purposes and potential benefits of the study in numerous meetings with the guardians of children in our study, many caregivers would regularly waylay the youth RAs when they came to visit and ask them pointed questions about what they were doing, why, what they got out of it, and what compensation the participants could expect. The study community largely misunderstood what research meant because their previous associations with "research" were really NGOs doing needs assessments to figure out how best to spend their charitable donations. Despite my earnest attempts to be clear from the beginning that I was an independent academic researcher and not someone representing any powerful or wealthy aid organizations, guardians' questions about compensation persisted because they associated research with aid. However, it also turned out that we had misunderstood their requests; through conducting the research itself, we eventually discovered that Josephine, the head teacher at the school, was giving people false information and making promises on my behalf in an effort to deflect attention from her own embezzlement of funds from a US church group—something we also would not have known had the youth RAs not asked probing questions. The resulting misinformation initially delayed the development of rapport with the families, but once we were in the know, we were able to remove all obfuscation.

I should point out that few of these challenges had to do directly with involving children and youth as opposed to a research team of adults. These issues are part of the broader dynamic of *studying down*, or studying a group of people less privileged than oneself, and could easily apply to any research project run by Westerners or even well-educated, upper-class Ugandans.

There are limits to participatory research with young people, however. The youth RAs enjoyed their involvement in research design, data collection, and analysis, but they clearly did not want to be involved in any writing up of the project; when I asked, they explicitly said that that was my job. It may be tempting to see this as a limitation, but as long as young people themselves determine the level of participation with which they are comfortable, participatory research still meets its objectives. Part of the point of doing participatory research is to give young people the opportunities to set their own boundaries, and even the youth RAs who were more academically inclined and endowed knew their own limitations in terms of being able to coauthor or even comment on the publication of the findings. So they were perfectly happy to leave that to me. For that reason, though, while the interpretation of the data was informed by input from the youth RA research team, the representation of the research in this volume is mine exclusively and therefore does not contain—nor should it be taken as containing—the definitive "voice" of children (James 2007, 264).

The Benefits of Participatory Research with Young People

Despite—or perhaps because of—the challenges associated with participatory research, I am confident that the involvement of young and old local stakeholders in the research enhanced the quality of the results. In the end, this participatory, collaborative design brought many benefits to various stakeholders of all ages; those benefits extended well beyond the research findings. Regular reflection with my research team helped build collaborative relationships between the children and the adults in the project as it progressed, and people learned more about themselves and one another in the process. Youth RAs said they had never realized how they themselves had been affected by orphanhood until they got to know the younger children; by the same token, the adults had never realized how children felt about their own circumstances until the project prompted them to ask—and listen. These secondary objectives of participatory research can thus end up becoming the most important advantages to participants, above and beyond the purposes of the study itself.

In this way, participatory ethnography actually becomes *transformative* of young people and their relationships with their communities as they realize that they have to work together across all ages to better meet the needs of OVC. Involving children and young people in research also yields greater ownership of knowledge production and organizational practice. By the end of fieldwork, youth RAs who were saying they never "had a heart" for young children before had taken a vested interest in mentoring the children in their study groups, and Faridah was emerging as an important leader in her community. This result should be no different for research than for the applied projects that come out of them: the project enabled youth RAs to network with other local stakeholders, receive training in marketable skills, and gain work experience. The study's youth RA research team also developed subsequent longer-term collaborations with the study community. For example, youth RAs and caregivers from the study transitioned into a local committee for an international NGO that provided employment to mostly female caretakers and improved educational opportunities for the neediest OVC from the study. Through this experience, youth RAs also learned to do cooperative needs assessments to help identify other potential beneficiaries in the community. Faridah is still working in this area as well.

Youth RAs were even able to carry forward a number of skills they learned into their careers as they got older. When I met with some of the youth RAs in July 2014, they each spoke of the way they have applied what they learned as youth RAs to their current activities. Michael and James, both working for telecom companies at the time, said they were essentially using research techniques they had learned as youth RAs to do market research.

Michael has also found his research experience useful in the youth group he is involved with in his own community. "Not most of us have gotten those chances," he pointed out. "[Employers] really enjoy if you have some experience behind you." He found it a distinct advantage when the youth group set about community organizing: "What you took us through, that taught me a lot because in most cases when [the youth group] used to convene . . . these guys [organizing with me] never knew anything about making focus groups, carrying out interviews, questionnaires, maybe drawing up notes. All they used to do is come in and sit around; they don't take notes." Michael thus felt better prepared to conduct activities that involved some basic research skills. Most important, his experience as a youth RA had taught him to listen and observe before jumping to conclusions—a lesson that came in handy for the purpose of community organizing: "Basically, you don't need to talk to the person but basically just look at a person; focus on a person, see how he acts, what he does." The techniques Michael learned from doing research with children (fig. 8) helped him "read" adults he encountered in his youth group work—not least because he had had to mediate the expectations of guardians during his research with children. As a result of his training, Michael knew how to approach people sensitively and could advise others in his community organizing team. He volunteered to interview people around the community and inform people about voluntary HIV counseling and testing. Because he was able to conduct focus groups about counseling without any further training, he gained valuable "participatory capital" (Wood 2013) with the organizers, who were, as Michael put it, "so, so, so, so, surprised!" that someone his age, from his community, and with his level of education possessed such skills.

James said he has had a similar experience: When the telecom company he was working for made him a sales representative and he was asked to conduct research about new market territory, he borrowed ideas from the youth RA training. For example, he said that to avoid being nervous when approaching retailers, he tried relating to them in the same way he had with the

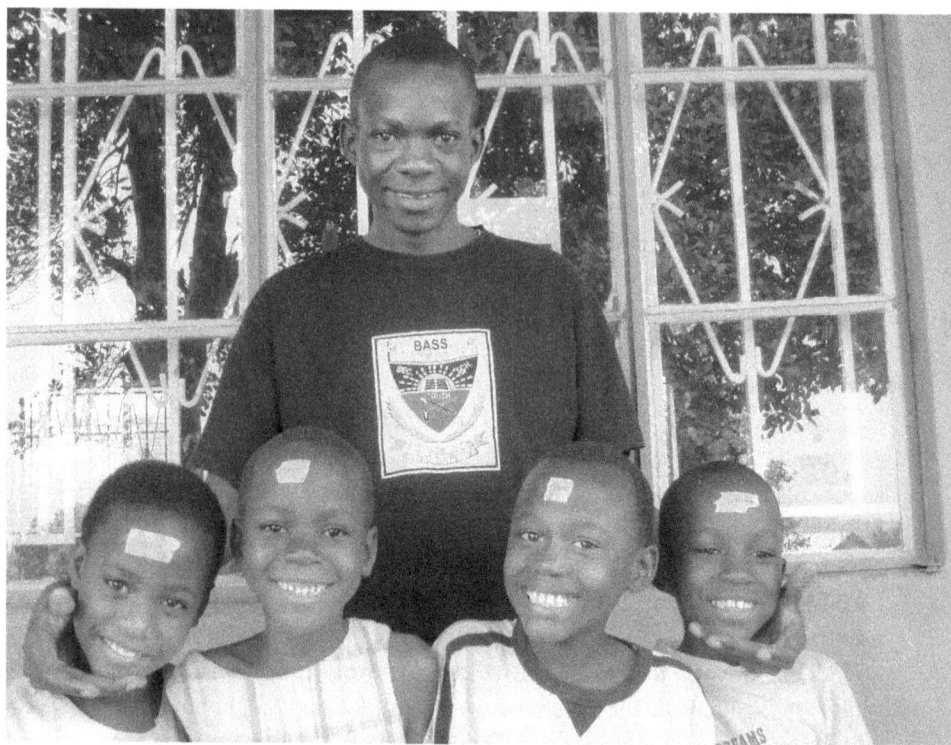

FIGURE 8. Youth research assistant Michael stands with his focus group children on the day they met in July 2007.

children during the research. "My target is being at par with each and every retailer who is selling our products," he said. "So I use the same idea: I go into someone's retail shop, I say 'I am so-and-so and I would like to know you.' So I relate those guys to kids . . . just transferring the small ideas that I had with kids to people I see in my work." James was actually assigned to do company outreach in the same area where we had conducted research, so he was already familiar with it, and he was able to employ data collection techniques in the marketing research: "I developed this system of recording. I remember when you gave us the voice recorder devices. When we're having a meeting, at least I have to record, go sit back, focus on what I heard. . . . I used not to do that, but through research training and those practices meeting those kids—jotting down ideas, writing notes, recording and then listening—I do it. So before I sleep at least I go to that idea; it's now in me and I like it." It has even helped him do better presentations: "At first I used to present reports in Excel sheets, but I once sent in a report using the PowerPoint presentations where there were slides and photos, and the managers were like, 'Wow, what a brilliant idea!'" James's colleagues even told him they wanted him to stop because it made them look bad, so that they had to work harder to keep up with him. But his manager said, "Go ahead and do what you're doing because we like this."

Jill, who had completed a bachelor's degree in development economics by 2014, found even more practical applications for the youth RA training: "Recently, I applied for a job, and one of its requirements was having done research. . . . You needed to have done a bit of research, especially with HIV-related issues, so I also attached my certificate we got from A-TRAIN." The others chimed in that the certificates of completion of the youth RA training, aside from signaling the achievement of a skill set, were important for building employment dossiers in Uganda. James even had his with him in his backpack, but it had gotten water-damaged. "That's why Mummy had ours laminated right away," Jill replied.

Just after graduation, Jill landed an internship at the national electricity authority, in a new consumer affairs unit. She quickly found herself advocating for participatory action research techniques similar to those she had employed as a youth RA:

> Initially, the CEO . . . wasn't sure if we should go down to the people to find out from the consumers how long they got power, when it got disconnected, etc. . . . My boss said, "Let's come up with ideas on how it will work." So I was like, "We can reach down! We can go to the people, we can organize awareness weeks, go to the community itself, ask these people what are the problems that [the electricity provider] causes when they come here—because these are the laws; this is what they are supposed to do—but what do they do here?"
>
> So I tried to apply that [youth RA training]. Actually, I came up with a few ideas about going to the people directly, giving out our number so that people contact us directly and we let them know what should happen besides what [the provider] tells them should happen. So actually, we did some small research—even we started awareness weeks, public hearing from community, down down to the people, because I knew it would work how we had done it before [in the research with children], reaching exactly to the people themselves rather than hearing [the distributor], who would tell us otherwise.

Michael added:

> The skills you taught us—because we learnt the visual research, the audio research . . . When you sit back home and get those reports you used to do, you look at the kids and the stories you used to write, and you're like, "Oh my God, I can't believe it was all me!" That's what basically I am so proud of because when I sit in a group in these CBOs [community-based organizations] and these guys are giving their ideas or their topic, once he says something I've

already at least gotten the broad [research] approach. I already know where it's going to end, and how he has started it, so at least I am telling them this is how we do it. Because that's what I'm involved in, still.

In fact, Michael thinks that in the CBO research they were conducting about HIV/AIDS in the community, they only scratch the surface without considering the broader context and the whole person. In our project, he learned to take the time to get to know the children and get relevant information in various ways that could benefit the CBO research as well. I was pleased that, although none of them chose social research as a career, they were still drawing on the skills we had taught them in their own ways—not only for their own betterment but also for that of the community.

Ethnographic Contributions to OVC Policy Analysis

The insights gained by employing former child research participants as youth RAs could not have been gained without the extended ethnographic inclusion of young people, as both participants and researchers. There were four primary benefits of using youth RAs. First, having older children who have "survived" orphanhood act as youth RAs speaks to concerns about young people's competency to conduct research; through their own life experience, language, and other cultural competencies, they were already poised to become successful junior "native" anthropologists. Second, the youth RAs regularly helped me resolve issues of representativeness. For instance, when a youth RA talked about a particular child's experience, I regularly asked the team to what extent they thought it was representative of other OVC's experiences—or children's experiences more broadly. Answers to such questions were usually qualified with nuances that furthered our common understandings of children's experiences and drove our research agenda in new directions. Third, the team members regularly drew on their own relatively recent childhoods to relate to the younger child participants and to reflect on their own responses to orphanhood. In this sense, it became a longitudinal study of orphans' experiences over time. Fourth, youth RAs helped discover that OVC themselves may have very different concerns and competencies than their caregivers and aid organizations often presume—some examples of which I will elaborate on in later chapters. A fifth, corollary benefit was that by participating in the study, youth RAs were able to process and articulate their own experiences of orphanhood in ways that they were unable to when they were younger participants in my previous study, which in turn gave them deeper perspectives on the situations of the children in their focus groups. Ethnography is a highly empathetic enterprise, and in this situation, the youth RAs came to feel deeply for the children with whom they worked—redoubling their dedication to the project and its goals to ameliorate the suffering of OVC like those they had gotten to know through their participation in the project.

Overall, such incidents indicated that community responses to AIDS orphanhood, often driven by both global and local assumptions about childhood, underestimated children's ability to comprehend disease and death, as well as their supposed resilience in the face of such adversities as the loss of parents. This study suggests that child-centered, participatory ethnographic research may yield more effective and sustainable policy and programming recommendations that reflect children's actual rather than assumed needs better than conventional research methods typically used in aid organizations' outcome-focused programming and assessment. The youth RAs were in a better position to elicit children's honest responses: Ugandan children tend to view adults as authority figures with privileged knowledge they impart to children—not the other way around. Children often aim to please adults by providing "correct" answers to questions, as pupils do to teachers. When it comes to orphanhood at the hands of AIDS in Uganda, however, the children who have experienced it are clearly the experts. They only needed to be made comfortable with the notion that they had something to contribute to adults' understandings, and here again is where ethnographic fieldwork—which involves extended stays and high levels of sustained involvement with a community to build rapport—proves effective for breaking down relationships of adult–child authority. This process can take some time for most adult researchers. For the youth RAs, however, building rapport with the younger children took no time at all: rather, the children in their focus groups took to them immediately, as "big brothers and sisters" in whom they could confide, ultimately providing the children with valuable counseling and mentorship.

Getting the Policy Makers to Listen

It is clear that organizations' need to demonstrate immediate results for funders drives a short-term, positivist, quantitative research agenda that makes it difficult to incorporate such techniques. As Andy West also points out, "A focus on process might dissipate the power structure and rationales for outputs and planning" (2007, 123). Again, it seems that ethnographic enquiry is especially appropriate to the task of refocusing organizational practice on process rather than measuring and outputs, which is what I strive for throughout this volume. Such a focus holds particular promise for children in difficult circumstances, many of whom are finding fewer and fewer adults on whom they can rely to help fulfill their needs. But because of the predominance of short-term funding cycles and quantitative performance measures, organizations can also find longitudinal, interpretivist research of less value—and despite purported belief in children's abilities, they may doubt the verity of data collected by young people.

In the absence of those who can provide for children's needs, however, their rights to participation take on incredible urgency. Participatory ethnography is a great way to start addressing the structures that prevent not only participation by children but the full realization of children's rights. In the process, youth RAs' feedback indicates, it also helps build young people's esteem and confidence. The youth RAs even identified ancillary benefits going back to being child participants in my previous research. Michael, reflecting on his initial participation as a twelve-year-old informant for *Pillars of the Nation* (Cheney 2007b), said, "It's now coming to more than twelve years since the first experience. Because I remember the first time you came to class. . . . It was a very, very nice experience because then you look back and you always think that that really boosted our esteem and gave us the confidence."

Jill agreed: "I also think it was more than research itself; it was more even us ourselves, like developing us. . . . It started everything: going to school and reaching where we are."

Policy makers truly wishing to make a lasting impact on children's lives would do well to consider these benefits.

The next several chapters draw primarily on the data collected by youth RAs to explore the impact of poverty, AIDS, and orphanhood on individual children, families, communities, and social institutions. I do so by detailing the longitudinal experiences of young people of various ages, including the youth RAs—most of whom grew up as orphans themselves—as well as incorporating the data they collected from younger children.

PART THREE

Orphanhood in the Age of HIV and AIDS

Orphanhood, Poverty, and the Post-ARV Generation

The youth research assistants (RAs) for this project were born around 1990, the year that HIV testing was introduced in Uganda. I conducted initial fieldwork with them in 2001, the year generic antiretroviral therapy (ART) made the treatment of HIV/AIDS available to a significant number of people (Whyte 2014, 6). Unfortunately, this treatment came too late for the parents of a number of them, who had already succumbed to AIDS by the time I met their children. By contrast, the children with whom they did research when they became youth RAs for this project from 2007 to 2009 had been born around 2001, when antiretrovirals (ARVs) were in wider use. Both cohorts thus fall into what I am calling the post-ARV generation. This chapter thus constitutes the first half of part 3 of the book, which provides a nuanced, longitudinal perspective on the post-ARV generation's experiences of orphanhood in the post-ARV era by discussing the lives of its earlier cohort.

It is important to note that while HIV/AIDS has certainly shaped the lives of the young people who became youth RAs for this project, the life stories in this chapter demonstrate that it is primarily *poverty* that continues to mark their experiences, influence their choices, and impinge on their chances in life. Aside from growing up in the era of HIV/AIDS, these children are also part of the "youth bulge" in population that has experienced the neoliberal retreat of the state, first under global economic restructuring and later under economic austerity. These factors all intersect to create the challenges and obstacles that shape young people's lives today.

In this chapter, I therefore bring attention to the daily struggles that young people have faced in the contemporary Ugandan context, where indeed *all* children are affected in some way by HIV/AIDS but also by persistent structural, household-level, and/or individual poverty. The youth RAs' stories also provide illustrative examples of the life trajectories of orphans and vulnerable children as well as insights into the resilience and survival strategies employed by young people throughout Africa. Their life stories are broadly indicative of the struggles of many Ugandan children to grow up, with or without their parents. Though the youth research assistants without parents continued to feel the sting of their parents' absence as they came of age, subsequent challenges of educational attainment, economic hardships, health, and family support also impinged on their daily lives throughout adolescence and young adulthood. While it is difficult to isolate HIV/AIDS as a cause of their suffering, these problems were often painfully amplified for the orphans. Further, they had certain gendered dynamics. However, access to resources and entitlements—particularly in the form of property and livelihood—was increasingly difficult for all of the youth research assistants to come by. Thus, extending the children's life history model I established in *Pillars of the Nation* (Cheney 2007b) to implement a longitudinal model for the study of young people's lives that in this case shows how orphanhood, HIV/AIDS, and poverty have intersected to affect this generation of young people over the life course. In the process, it also reveals how I as an engaged researcher have become entwined with them and their families over the years as research subjects, participants, beneficiaries, social kin, and coresearchers. The rapport gained through this experience thus provides a better understanding of what makes us a research team. All names in the chapter are pseudonyms.

Sumayiya: The Struggles of a Female Double Orphan

Sumayiya's experiences serve as an example of how double orphanhood can impact girls in particularly compromising ways. Sumayiya had had a difficult childhood in which she had lost her father at the age of six and floated with her mother from one relationship to the next. Her school attendance was sporadic at best; by the age of eleven she had been out of school for a year and a half. After encountering abuse and neglect at the hands of her mother and her mother's many subsequent boyfriends, Sumayiya finally ran away to resume her education. When I met her, she was fourteen and in the fifth grade. She was living with an aunt who was a doctor and was putting her through school. She had hoped to be a lawyer so she could help children like her attain their rights.

I had kept in touch with Sumayiya throughout my absence from Uganda, and I had been worried about her and her own survival strategies, with good reason. I learned from our occasional e-mail communication that she had left her uncle and aunt's house after some older boys staying there were "trying to do things" to her. "But I was too young," she told me, "so when you e-mailed me telling me to get to someplace safe, I left without saying anything to anybody. No one from that place bothered about me or came to look for me, but I spent most of my childhood there, so I went back and later told my aunt why I left." Sumayiya said her aunt showed no reaction to her allegations toward the boys, but they agreed it was for the best that she had left. She entered a boarding school, where I helped her with fees.

I was therefore eager to catch up with Sumayiya in the summer of 2007. Research coordinator Faridah and I met her at a restaurant in town. She came through the door in jeans and a flowing white blouse. She looked much thinner in the face and yet shapelier than when I had last seen her in 2001 at fourteen. Now twenty, she had grown into quite a strong young lady. We hugged tightly, touching cheeks on both sides. She was noticeably distressed despite her excitement at seeing me again, and she kept quiet until Faridah had left. Then she explained to me why she had not reported back to school when the semester had started a few weeks earlier; it was not because I had delayed with her fees but because she had had a boyfriend she had met in high school before the O-level exams. "I messed up," she said as she held back tears. I had a feeling this was coming, but I listened patiently as she revealed that she had gotten pregnant. The school had found out near the end of the previous term, and they had said they would have to notify her guardian, but she said she had none, and "You were far away," so they told her she could not report for the new term. Despite a teen pregnancy rate of 25 percent in Uganda, the government policy at the time was to expel girls who got pregnant.[1] Girls (unlike the boys who impregnate them) are often excluded from school on the assumption that they will negatively influence other students, so they are not only expelled but are expelled in a public and shaming manner to make them a deterrent to other students. It can drive many girls to seek abortions to avoid the stigma. "I couldn't abort," Sumayiya explained, "but I really messed up. I just wanted to see you straightaway because I did not want to lie about it." She was afraid I would be mad at her, but that was one of the last emotions I felt at that moment; I was just concerned for her and hated to see more doors close to her just as she had managed to open them. Though there was no legal prohibition against young mothers returning to school to complete their educations, it is really up to individual school administrators to decide how to handle such situations. Because of the public humiliation of expulsion, the stigma of teenage motherhood among the educated, and the lack of support by teachers and schools, few girls go back to school after giving birth. Even where girls are allowed to resume their studies after giving birth, their ability to attend school depends on the support of the schools and relatives who can help care for their children while they study; Sumayiya had neither.

I asked Sumayiya if she had been to see a doctor, but she said she had not, even though she guessed that she was about four months into her pregnancy. She was primarily reluctant because she knew she would be tested for HIV as part of the efforts in prevention of mother-to-child transmission (PMTCT). As I mentioned in part 1, a large part of Uganda's success in combating HIV infection has been through PMTCT (Whyte 2014). For this reason, an HIV test is a mandatory first step in prenatal treatment. It is thus also often when women first discover their HIV status. For this reason, Eva Vernooij and Anita Hardon (2013) have critiqued this policy's implications for the consent of pregnant women like Sumayiya, who may *not* want to be tested but who must submit to it if they want to receive prenatal and postnatal services. Further, she was no longer together with the father, but Sumayiya said she had told him about the child and he said would support him or her (once the baby was born, however, he refused to acknowledge it was even his)—yet she did not want to involve him in things like doctor's visits. I told her that if she wanted me to, I would go with her to the hospital.

Sumayiya's pregnancy was just another knot in a string of already complex problems and challenges: Sumayiya's mother had passed away in 2006. She apparently suffered a painful death from a liver condition that swelled her stomach. Sumayiya had not seen her mother in years, but when she received the news that her mother was sick, she found out where she lived and went to her. They were able to see each other before she passed, and they made amends. In fact, her mother was only happy to see her, and Sumayiya cared for her until she died.

Afterward, Sumayiya discovered that her relatives had taken her eight-year-old half-brother Alan all the way back to his estranged father's home village in Kanungu, in far western Uganda. On New Year's Day, she went to fetch him and brought him to live with her and her roommate Evelyn, whom she had met at school. Sumayiya employed a common orphan coping mechanism of relying on her peer social network for support in the absence of relatives. Evelyn, who also had few family members on whom to fall back, had completed secondary school the previous year with the help of sponsorship, and the three of them shared a room. Sumayiya and Evelyn had managed to start a small clothing business in Owino Market, one of East Africa's largest outdoor markets and a mouse maze of makeshift kiosks. They would buy dresses from secondhand bundles, wash and iron them, and then hang them in their stall for resale. The business helped bring in a bit of income, and Evelyn watched Alan while Sumayiya was at school. They had enrolled him in a Universal Primary Education school, but it still cost about 30,000 Uganda shillings (UGX), or about 18 US dollars (USD), in materials fees that they struggled to collect, so his attendance was uneven as he was dismissed whenever these fees were not paid.

Having left school in 2007, then, Sumayiya thought she might instead go for a diploma in computer administration that could land her a good office job. She seemed to have thought it out well, and considering her situation, I figured it was probably for the best. She could complete the first course in three months, then have her baby, and see about completing the next course in six months. She figured she could still work at the market part-time while she went to the computer school, and Evelyn, whom she described as a "sister," agreed to continue to help her with Alan and her new baby. I was impressed with her resilience; I told her I would help her with the computer training fees if she felt she could cope up with the whole situation (and she said she could). She expressed interest in still helping with my research in return. Given her own harrowing experience with orphanhood and her strong character, I thought she would do well as a youth research assistant for this study, but being pregnant and having so many other responsibilities might prevent it. We would just have to wait and see how it would go.

Malik: Family as Both a Help and a Hindrance

Although Malik was also a double orphan, his experiences differed greatly from Sumayiya's, partly due to a more stable extended-family support and his own talents, and also because of his gender. But his upbringing was still not without its challenges, and some of his family's efforts to support him might well have backfired without additional support.

Malik was raised by his grandmother, who figured out early on that his talent for music would help him in life. After his parents died, she had put him in contact with people who might be able to cultivate his musical skills, and those skills would help him get an education. Back in primary school, he had fallen in well with Mr. Kisakye, the music teacher who ran a dance troupe that was often hired for entertainment at public functions. His participation in the troupe allowed him to earn income from an early age, but the family still struggled to meet his increasing school fees, and they asked me to assist them.

After arriving in Uganda in 2007, I started making some calls and reached Alex, Malik's young uncle, who insisted on meeting with me before leading me to Malik. It turned out that Alex may have had other motives in getting to me before I talked to Malik, however; Alex had always tried to control the school fees I sent for Malik, and I had been growing suspicious. He claimed that he could not pay the school directly, and I had not understood why. I had thought he was on some kind of partial music scholarship at a prestigious high school and that I was merely paying the remainder of his fees. But when I returned in 2007, Alex explained that he was a good friend of the music teacher at Malik's school. Alex had discussed his struggles paying for his grandmother's rent and still getting Malik through school and asked what his friend could do to help. They decided that the teacher would claim Malik as a dependent so he could use the teachers' tuition discount for relatives. This, Alex claimed, was how he was actually able to pay about a third less than the regular tuition. Alex said that the school took the fees out of the teacher's pay, so they gave the teacher the money for Malik's tuition directly instead of paying the bursar at the school. That is what he had actually meant by "music scholarship."

This explanation too turned out to be an elaborate lie. I tried to be sure that Malik was always involved in the transfer of his own school fees by transferring the money in Alex's name (the company through which I sent the money had a minimum age for pick-up, and Malik was still too young at the time), but I sent a separate e-mail to Malik with the password, so that they effectively had to go collect the money together with the two pieces of information. However, I learned later that Alex had hacked Malik's e-mail account to get hold of the password himself. Having incurred some bad debt, Alex took all of Malik's fees one term in 2008 and ran off to Kenya with it.

In chapter 2, I already referred to how orphan targeting for aid or charity was having adverse effects on children and families, and I will expand on how orphanhood is affecting families in chapter 7, but Malik and Alex's example illustrates how orphans and the assistance they receive can be exploited—even by trusted members of their own families. His grandmother and aunties did their best to mediate as well as compensate for Alex's wrongdoing, but the incidence strained Malik's relationship with Alex (not to mention my relationship with Alex) and continues to do so to this day: Malik was livid to learn of Alex's deception and siphoning off of resources meant to secure Malik's education.

I was able to meet with Malik a few days after seeing Alex on my return in 2007. He still looked much the same, though he had grown by about two feet. His voice had also changed, obviously. I called Sumayiya while I was with Malik, and she briefly talked to him, as she had gone to grade school with him but had not seen him since. She commented on Malik's deepened voice as well. Malik was living with the traditional dance troupe to which he belonged. It had a nice, quiet compound (when they were not all banging on drums) not far from Makerere University's bustling main gate. About seventeen boys stayed there in a dorm that resembled a shipping container, but the main house was nearly empty except for a room that housed all of their instruments and another that housed the troupe's office. They rehearsed in the main room when it rained. An attendant took us through and even gave us a newsletter from 2005 that highlighted their performance for President Museveni at a prayer breakfast. The troupe was also slated to dance for dignitaries at the Commonwealth Heads of Government Meeting that was hosted in Uganda in 2007.

According to the newsletter, the dance troupe got many of its young members—boys and girls—from the streets. It even put them back in school and had them complete their studies while they were performing with the troupe. After Malik became a regular fixture in the group, his grandmother recommended he go to stay with the troupe to avoid the cost and hassle of moving across town every day. The troupe members practiced Monday, Wednesday, and Friday evenings and on weekends whenever they did not have shows. Though it was hostel-style living, there seemed to be decent discipline, and Malik seemed really happy there. He showed us even more newsletters with pictures of him and a short written piece about him. It mentioned that he was elected prefect of his house after only one term at the school. It struck me that Malik, also a double orphan, was doing so much better than other children in his situation, but then he had family and his musical community looking out for him, and despite his uncle's duplicitousness, his musical talent had helped him get by.

Malik's musical career would eventually take him even as far as South Korea to perform, but he still struggled to keep himself with enough work to make ends meet. He had wanted to go for a computer technology degree, but he did not have the funds, and anyway, he only wanted to do that on the spurious assumption that it would get him a job. He knew little about computers and, at the time, was doing better financially than the other youth research assistants, making an income through performing around town. But his music income was inconsistent at best; well into his twenties, he still stayed with his aunt who ran a restaurant in town. She felt maybe she was doing him no favors by coddling him, so in 2014, they decided he would go to Dubai to seek work. A lot of young Ugandan men were going there at the time, as there were plenty of jobs in construction, retail, and security for foreign laborers. He called me once in early 2015 to say he had gotten a job at a shoe store and was working ten to twelve hours a day while living in a tiny room in an apartment with other immigrants. "I now know the value of work," he assured me.

Though Malik had a lot of family support and his musical talents had taken him a long way, he essentially started working at a younger age than the other youth research assistants—albeit in a less hazardous occupation than many other children—and through that work was able to finish secondary school. As a young adult, however, he had to migrate to find enough work to afford the possibility of saving enough money to form his own household. Despite supposed economic growth, young Africans and orphans in particular are commonly driven to precarious forms of work such as migrant labor, sometimes knowingly and sometimes unwittingly, as returning to Sumayiya's example further illustrates.

Sumayiya, Again: Precarious Work, Precarious Relationships

I was supposed to meet Sumayiya at her place for lunch, but since she and Malik had attended primary school together and he expressed some excitement at the possibility of seeing her, I called to ask if we could come for lunch together. She said it was all right, so we (Alex, too) went together to Kasubi. One of my hosts had earlier expressed surprise that I was going there because it apparently had a reputation for being a tough neighborhood. Sumayiya met us at the gas station across the street from the *matatu* (shared minibus shuttle) stop (wearing a smock dress that hid her swelling belly) and brought us back behind a nursery school that masked a block of disheveled one-room apartments with no plumbing or electricity. She led us into the door of her one-room apartment. It was small, but it was clean, and the walls were painted a cheerful sky blue. There was a single queen bed and an armoire with a mirror. She, her roommate Evelyn, and her brother Alan all slept there. By the time Sumayiya later had her baby, Evelyn had left for work in Kenya, and she had asked Sumayiya to share the place with her young friend who was escaping an abusive relationship. Evelyn's friend had an eighteen-month-old girl, making a total of five people in the one-room apartment. They bought another foam mattress and placed that on the floor at night so everyone had a place to sleep.

I met her brother Alan, who seemed really reticent and sullen, perhaps because of his mother's fairly recent death. Like many boys I met, Alan seemed to radiate anger in his loss. Sumayiya told us about her shop and her interest in the computer course as she wandered in and out to cook. She served us a ton of food, and we had a nice lunch together before I had to move on. We would meet again soon to pay her computer course fees and go for prenatal care.

*

By the time I returned in December 2007, Sumayiya had delivered a healthy baby girl and named her Priscilla after a character in a novel. She tried contacting the father again, but he could not be bothered. Priscilla was three months old and just learning to smile when I got there, and many friends had given me baby clothes to bring for her. "She is somehow a comfort," Sumayiya confessed.

"How do you mean?"

"She helps me to not feel so lonely," she said as she beamed at her bubbly little girl.

When I returned again in 2009 to finish the orphan study, Sumayiya had finished her computer degree. She was still having trouble finding work, however, as she had few connections to people who worked in offices, and in Kampala it is certainly about *who* you know. It did not help her financial situation that Owino Market burned down in early 2009. Sumayiya was no longer keeping her stall with her friends, but she had been working for a woman who rented a secondhand clothing stall there, in which she managed to add a few of her own pieces. So when the market went up in flames, so did her meager investments.

Despite Sumayiya's apparent lack of social capital and her subsequent reliance on precarious work, she did not give up trying to attain the training to enter the formal labor market: At about the time of the Owino fire, she heard from a friend that there were good prospects in nursing, so she decided to switch gears and try to get a nursing diploma. This decision was made partly on the assumption that her aunt, who is a doctor, could help her get a job—even though they had not spoken much since Sumayiya had left her aunt's house.

Where Sumayiya lacked kin connections for support, she sought support through other social relationships, which also put her at risk of exploitation. She had started a precarious relationship in late 2008 with a young Ugandan man living in Denmark whom she had met while he was home on holiday. He quickly gained her favor by helping her move to a better apartment, but he was not gaining her trust. "The thing with him," she confided to me in January 2009, "is that he cheats—but he says he is serious." Needless to say, this assertion raised an immediate red flag. I pursued the topic and found out that despite his having been in town for only three weeks on his most recent holiday, she had caught him sleeping around. Yet, as a young mother with no one else to rely on, she realized that he offered her valuable financial assistance. And he had promised to take her away from it all by bringing her to Denmark. They had already applied for a fiancée visa, and Sumayiya was preparing to leave Alan and Priscilla with her brother's wife so she could go, "just to earn a little money and then come back." Instantly, images of Sumayiya getting sold into sex slavery flooded my imagination. It sounded far-fetched to her, but I knew that young, single mothers struggling to support their children were particularly vulnerable to being sex-trafficked, lured by a sweet talker promising love, support, and easy money doing menial jobs abroad.[2] I also knew that Sumayiya was exactly the kind of girl to whom this happened, and it happened in exactly the way she was describing. Having grown up without a father or other strong male role models, Sumayiya seemed easily drawn to men who showed her the slightest kindness, repeating her mother's patterns of male dependency by finding partners willing and able to support her and her dependents. Even if trafficking was a worst-case scenario, I knew that this could not end well. I told her so, and I worked hard to wean her of the idea that she needed a boyfriend who could not even be faithful for three weeks; it was a financial relief at the time, but she would end up paying dearly, one way or another. Even after she found out that he had slept with the new neighbor within a few days of moving her into her new apartment, she still held out hope that he might change—another idea of which I and other members of our research team worked hard to dissuade her. I encouraged her to try to make it on her own by bringing her a new laptop and hiring her to do some archival work for me. I had also found Alan educational assistance after his father died in 2008, and I helped her go to nursing school when she decided that computer administration was not for her. Still, she secretly pursued the fiancée visa. When her application was denied, however, the guy immediately dropped her—to my relief.

That was not the end of Sumayiya's vulnerability to potential exploitation, though. After she got her nursing diploma, Sumayiya managed to open a small dispensary. She occasionally contacted me by e-mail or through Facebook and was seemingly doing well. But a lot of young Ugandans like Malik and Sumayiya are lured by promises of greener pastures and easy money abroad. In 2011, I suddenly got a Facebook message that she was in Malaysia. At first, I thought maybe it was a hoax, but I was able to verify that it was her by probing about some confidential information. She said she had gone there through a Nigerian boyfriend who paid part of her fees to go to nursing school there. He was being abusive, though, and she could not leave because the university had her passport and would not give it back while she still had a balance on her tuition. I found this highly suspect: schools do not hold students' passports as collateral against tuition payments.

At the same time, she was posting pictures of herself wearing tight, skimpy dresses in big shopping malls or in the back of expensive cars with leather interiors. The occasional much older, white male "friend" popped up in her pictures, too. Around the same time, the *Washington Post* broke a story about the Ugandan government negotiating the release of twenty-one trafficked women in Malaysian police custody.[3] They had uncovered a trafficking ring run by Nigerians, who promised Ugandan women lucrative cleaning jobs or schooling opportunities. By March 2012, Sumayiya was still in Malaysia, although she said she had left the abusive boyfriend, was living with some other African women, and was working in an African restaurant. Meanwhile, the United Nations reported that about six hundred Ugandan women had been trafficked to Malaysia.

Just as suddenly, Sumayiya wrote that she was able to make her way back to Uganda in April 2012, but no one else was able to confirm that for me, and when I said I was coming to Uganda in July 2012, she said she was looking forward to seeing me but was evasive about giving me her contact information. Faridah and I both failed to locate her, despite going to her old home, friends' homes, and her places of business. Just before I left, she wrote me a message saying we would unfortunately miss each other because she got an opportunity through another friend to go to South Africa and had to leave in a rush. This seemed unlikely, her having just gotten back from Malaysia—and when questioned later, she said that she didn't actually go to South Africa. She may just have been avoiding us. In any case, she provided the number of the relative watching Alan and Priscilla and encouraged me to contact them so I could see the children. But given the circumstances, I thought it better to wait and see them when Sumayiya was also there.

Initially, I was very worried about Sumayiya, whom I considered very sweet but a bit naive and vulnerable to exploitation, particularly by young men whom she hoped would love and care for her. But I gradually realized that she had become a grown woman making decisions with a clear idea of the risks and consequences of her actions. Roy Huijsmans and Simon Baker (2012) have critiqued certain child trafficking discourses that empty young people of their agency and their avid desires to move abroad in search of work. Like so many young women, Sumayiya through her story bears the mark of recent neoliberal influences on the aspirations of disadvantaged youth (Swift and Maher 2008). Media images depicting the relative freedom, independence, and wealth of a life abroad lead young women like Sumayiya to make certain calculated risks, especially when it comes to romantic entanglements (M. Hunter 2010). When it does not work out as they had hoped, many young women often have to rescue themselves from the undesirable consequences. I realized that there was nothing I could do to protect Sumayiya anymore, since she was now an adult making her own decisions; I could only be her sympathetic ear when she was ready to tell me about it.

That time did not come until 2015, when she got in touch with me again over Facebook and expressed interest in seeing me when I was in town next. I had traveled to Kampala many times in the previous several years, but

Sumayiya had not resurfaced, and I had given up trying to see her. This time, however, she made an appointment with me and actually kept it. She showed up to lunch one day, dressed more like a soccer mom than a streetwalker. In tow was a reticent young man she introduced as her boyfriend and business partner (and who may or may not be Priscilla's father). He said not a word and barely looked up from his cell phone as Sumayiya and I spent several hours getting caught up. Faridah was anxious to see her, too, so the three of us had dinner together a few days later. Sumayiya recounted the story of the abusive Nigerian boyfriend in Malaysia—but she also told us about the Singaporean businessman who brought her across the border to have her work for him in his shop, and the German investor who sent her to Shanghai to go to trade shows with his Chinese contacts to figure out what products she could import from China to sell in Uganda. The German investor ultimately sent her back home, and there she was selling thermoses for him in Kampala.

Faridah and I were finding a lot of this story far-fetched, but Sumayiya did show us pictures on her phone of her and her Chinese counterparts at trade shows in Shanghai. In any case, we were glad that she was back home safe and seemed to be holding her own.

James: Never Giving Up on Education

Another youth research assistant who seemed to be holding his own despite multiple setbacks was James. James's story exemplifies the struggles of intergenerational poverty exacerbated by orphanhood but also the hope of overcoming it with hard work and a persistent determination to attain an education. It also provides an example of what happens to a household that suddenly loses its primary breadwinner. The death of his father in 2001 had severely limited James's ability to continue with his education (Cheney 2007b, 98), but James had not given up: he was able to finish primary school after his father had passed away while he was in sixth grade, and because he was such an exceptional student, he received partial tuition remission from a nearby secondary school. But even then, his mother had trouble finding fees for him because she did not work, James and his brother Alex were in the same class, and she also had other children finishing school. The family kept delaying with the payments until the school chased away James and Alex in their third year of high school. Even then, James came back to take final exams and got the fifth highest scores in the class. Their mother had given up even trying to pay fees, yet James and Alex both expressed an avid desire to continue to go to school, so they moved to a cheaper school that was a bit farther away. There they completed high school, but they still had problems paying the fees, so the school sent them away in the last term to another school to prepare for the O-level exit exams. James did quite well, though he had been in and out of school the whole year. He was out of school the entire last term, in fact, but he would sit in the library and copy notes from his friends. When he took the exam at the end of the year, he got several distinctions, including a first distinction in physics. They could find no other scholarships, though, so at that point his mother told him she just could not manage to pay the fees for him to continue schooling to A levels (college prep, mirroring the British school system of O-level classes followed by A-level classes prior to university enrollment). Aside from school fees, they had shifted from the rental house where they moved in 2001 after his father died, which cost 30,000 UGX (about 18 USD) per month, to a house that cost 50,000 UGX (30 USD). James's mother ran a small convenience store out of the house, selling some necessities to the local community. But even that income combined with the money James's older sister contributed from her teaching job did not bring in enough to support everyone in the household, including James, his three brothers, and their little nephew, his sister's child. Although James did well on the exams, he owed 220,000 UGX (110 USD) in back fees to the school, so his exam results and certificate were withheld by the school until he paid the debt. He could not go on to A-level classes, in any case, until he got his certificate.

A number of monographs about urban children and youth in Africa have shown how the belief that educational attainment as a means out of poverty has led families to make incredible sacrifices to send their children through school (Honwana and Boeck 2005; Cole and Durham 2008; Hansen 2008; Mains 2013). And yet youth unemployment rates tell a different story: although sub-Saharan Africa was less affected by the global financial crisis than other regions were, youth unemployment still lingers at around 15 percent, and job creation has only slowed as a result (International Labour Office 2012). While his older siblings managed to find occasional work and chipped in to help their mother pay the rent, James still wanted to stay in school because he thought would have a better chance of getting a job if he had an A-level diploma. So he went to work in construction to try to raise his own fees. He would work the whole day at backbreaking tasks, digging trenches or hauling cement, and get only 1,000 UGX, the going rate for a bottle of soda at the time. It was obviously not enough to save for fees or rent. He said he had looked into going to an affordable Kampala secondary school where he heard there was a good science program. The number one student in the national A-level exams was from there that year, and James told me that if you came in number one in your class in overall exam results, the school would waive your tuition the following year. The fees were 260,000 UGX (130 USD) to start (with uniform and materials) and 120,000 UGX (70 USD) thereafter. His sister, who was teaching primary school in Masaka while their mother looked after her toddler, even promised him that she could get him half the money. But he still thought he had a shot at achieving the number one position and so might be retained on scholarship for his A-level classes. Even if he did not get a scholarship, I thought it was an affordable and wise investment, as James was an exceptionally bright student. I offered to help him with the other half of the fees so he could finish his A-level courses and exams.

As for the current research project, he liked the idea of becoming a youth research assistant, but it seemed to have stung when I mentioned that it would be a study of orphanhood. I got the sense he was still missing his father quite a bit, but I did not broach the subject just yet. He did seem to respond well to the idea that it would be therapeutic for both the older and the younger children.

As with the others, unexpected economic shocks and illness made life difficult for James. Later in 2007, his mother's convenience store was broken into and all her inventory stolen. In June 2008, James got sick with a cough, fever, and chest pains. He came down with ulcers and tuberculosis, probably due to the stress and crowded conditions where he was living. He wrote in a letter:

> The cough continued until when I started coughing blood. This was serious and my brother got some money and we went to the hospital. The doctor took some examinations on my chest and wrote to us [a prescription for] the medicine. Unfortunately, the money we had gone with was not enough. I got some of the medicine. After a week, the blood stopped. By then, I was not going to school. I used to stay in bed the whole day. Ulcers attacked me too. But I had this problem some time back. In that week a friend informed me that some exams were going to start. In pain I walked to school for a week, and I completed the exams . . . Mummy just looked at me because she had no money. When I told her to take me for treatment she replied, "We need to pay the house rent yet I have no money. You can even see my business is down." Truly, Kristen, we are in a poverty situation. I have now taken a month and some weeks at home.

I sent him some more money so he could get medical treatment. He had to stay in isolation, though, so again he was unable to go to school—and since he was told especially to avoid young children and old people, who are particularly susceptible to contracting the airborne disease, it precluded any visits to his study group for a while. I accompanied him to his study children's homes when he finally returned after an eight-month treatment regimen. The children were thrilled to see him, especially Belinda, who ran into his arms.

James continued his recovery over the course of several years, and with financial assistance, he managed to finish his A-level courses and exams. While his grades were still very good, they were not quite good enough to earn him a university scholarship. However, he very quickly managed to find work in a small Internet café. When I caught up with James again in 2012, he was doing quite well; he had gotten a marketing job with a leading cell phone company, and though he was still living at home with his mother, he took pride in being able to help her and his siblings with household expenses.

Since then, James has really come into his own; he completed his bachelor of science degree in computer information systems in 2015 while he was working and has advanced in the telecom company, and he met a young woman whom he wants to marry as soon as he has saved enough to build a house. There is hardly a vestige of the shy boy he used to be; he is now confident and focused on these goals, and he knows what steps he must take to reach them. We regularly meet when I come to Kampala. In March 2016, he asked me when the book was coming out and reminded me that he would need me to bring him a copy.

In sum, James's faith in schooling managed to help him to some extent, but persistent poverty after the loss of his father caused severe disruptions in James's education. Though he did not go as far as he might have, he was able to overcome these challenges through decent employment but mainly a determination to make it out of poverty.

Jill and Michael: Struggling against the Mathematics of Poverty

The Obonyo family serves as a contrast to orphaned children's experiences because Jill and Michael are the two youth research assistants who had *not* lost their parents. Even with both parents alive and well, though, many children have to struggle with similar grips of poverty. Jill and Michael's lives thus outwardly showed little contrast with double orphans like Sumayiya and Malik or single orphans like James. One could argue that they were doing much better in that the children were not required to work or find their own means of support, but their family struggled with the lack of social services available to keep them from going under. If we do the math, we see that young people in poor families, despite having one another for support, still struggle to break out of intergenerational poverty.

Jill wanted to be a judge when she was in sixth grade in 2001. In 2007, Jill still lived with her parents, brother, and sister in a cramped home in Namuwongo, a low-rent community of mostly northern Ugandan migrants to the city, but she had gotten into a rather prestigious boarding secondary school.

I caught up with Jill and her mother, Margaret, soon after I arrived in the summer of 2007. Margaret had been working for about a year for a cleaning company subcontracted to clean the Uganda Court of Appeals building. The government said it had no money to pay support staff, and thus government agencies were told to contract out the work. The contracted companies took the money but then kept the employees off the books and gave them a fraction of the money as salary. So the company employees worked very hard in an unstable job market for little pay. To feed her three children, Margaret got up early to walk two hours to work (taking *matatus* would cost 1,200 UGX [about 72 cents US] round-trip and would thus take too much out of her pay). There, she opened and cleaned the court chambers. After sessions started, she was sent to fetch judges and barristers their lunches, sodas, and tea. At the end of the day, Margaret and her coworkers tidied up, and she walked two hours back home. At the end of the month, she was given 90,000 UGX (about 54 USD). She mentioned that since her husband Vittore had fallen ill when the children were young, he had not been able to work much, and it stung his pride. The couple used to have a small convenience store adjacent to their house (which was originally built as a garage), but when the government hiked electricity rates, they were not able to maintain it, so they rented it out to someone to live in instead. They were also renting rooms in the house, but they eventually decided to stop after a while because they had two daughters, and Margaret was worried about the possibility of her daughters' "defilement" by single men to whom they might rent.[4] "I see it all the time at the courthouse," she told me. So they were making do with her job and the one rental, which pulled in 30,000 UGX (about 18 USD) per month.

That meant that the five of them (their daughter Michelle was eleven years old and in sixth grade, so she was still benefiting from universal primary education) subsisted on the equivalent of 72 USD per month. The World Bank defines living on less than 1 USD per day as absolute poverty. So my assistance with Jill and Michael's school fees enabled them to go to boarding schools, which was all that was keeping the children from experiencing the type of "poverty situation" James had described experiencing on a daily basis. Margaret had said she even had problems feeding the children when they were home on holiday because her salary was not enough and they had no land in Kampala on which to cultivate any crops. Vittore often went to his home village in Lira, where he had some land from which he could harvest staple foods, but even that could be insufficient. Such food insecurity is not uncommon for the urban poor.

We went to pay Jill and Michael's school fees and have the slips stamped. They were each 465,000 UGX (about 279 USD), but the schools also do a lot of nickel-and-diming to get more out of students, with additional money demanded for required school supplies (not just for the individual student but items like toilet paper, brooms, and mops for the whole school; their costs totaled about two weeks of Margaret's pay), field trips, and "workshops" during holidays. Despite the Obonyos' incredible sense of privilege at keeping the children in boarding school, they were well aware that access alone did not guarantee future economic stability. Schools themselves, whose reputations are riding on the success of their students in national exams, tend to implement draconian discipline and cultivate cutthroat competition between their students to achieve better results. Jill's school was strict, but that strictness apparently paid off when some of its students scored high enough on national exams to send them to the university on government scholarships. Parents were not even allowed to see their children outside of one Saturday visitation per month. Margaret had to talk with the deputy headmaster several times to gain permission for my visit. Even when we pulled up at the gate and the guard greeted us, however, he expressed skepticism that Jill would be let out of class to see us. But they called her and she came running and screaming. She gave me a big hug, and we barely avoided tears. Her face still looked the same, but she was about a foot taller. I had last seen her at age eleven, and now she was seventeen.

At A-levels, students concentrate in four subjects, though they still take others. Jill chose history, economics, divinity, and entrepreneurship—an interesting but not uncommon combination. Jill also told me about her daily eighteen-hour schedule. She and her classmates would get up at 4:00 a.m. for breakfast at 4:30 a.m., study hall from 5:00 to 7:00 a.m., classes from 7:00 a.m. to 5:00 p.m., time from 5:00 to 7:00 p.m. to take a shower, eat dinner, and do laundry, and then evening study hall from 7:00 to 10:00 p.m. The official schedule occupied virtually every minute of the day, presumably to keep children from goofing off. But students worked so hard that sometimes, Jill said, after 10:00 p.m. bedtime, they would sleep for only a few hours and then wake up at 2:00 a.m. to do some extra studying. This was not atypical of Uganda boarding school students, and their dedication to an institutional promise whose fulfillment was tenuous at best mystified me.

The school was strict indeed: Jill told me that there were about 300 students in the S5 class (roughly equivalent to junior year of US high school) but that there were only about 170 slots in S6 (senior year), so if she did not study hard, she might not get a place the following year. Or, she might be chased away for not buttoning the top button of her uniform or for letting her socks slouch too much. She told me that if people acted up in class, teachers often lined them up and caned the whole bunch, no questions asked. Schools are particularly authoritarian regimes, and despite my support of the children's efforts to be educated, I had to wonder whether it was all worth it, when most of these children would likely graduate from high school, and some also from university, to no job at all. But Jill and her mother agreed that it was better to be there on campus than at home. Like James with his faith in education, the Obonyos also believed in its ability to lift them from poverty. Margaret said, "Even when they are hungry or want a new shirt, I tell them, 'Concentrate on education first! Kristen is putting a bank there in your head, and that is the most important thing for your future.'" Margaret also recognized ancillary benefits for the children on campus: she mentioned that they were fortunate to be in such a nice environment, where the lawns that offer a far-off view of the city were well manicured and the air was clear, unlike in the dusty, smoggy city. "I hate the city campuses that are so cramped," Margaret muttered. "Me, if I had a compound [yard] like this one, I could stay there all day. It's not like our place where there is house after house and no grass. You should come [to] that side and see how full it is now!" I had visited their home many times during my stay in Uganda in 2000–2001, and it was indeed already cramped then, with few gardens and many challenges to accessing clean water, sanitation, and waste management. Such conditions had caused James to contract tuberculosis.

Despite their struggles, Jill seemed well adjusted. Having two parents who cared for her despite their severe financial limitations, she lived in an environment that was obviously much more stable than that of Sumayiya, who was a double orphan. Jill graduated from secondary school in 2009 with high marks and managed to get a full-tuition scholarship to study development economics at Makerere University. At about the same time, Margaret managed to land a contracted government job in Masaka that would provide her with better pay as well as benefits. She worked there for several years before managing to get a transfer back to Kampala so she could stay with her family. Jill graduated and managed to get an internship with an energy company —but she could not land a paying job and so moved back home with her parents. In 2014, she was working in a travel agency but still looking for something better.

After visiting Jill, we went to see her older brother, Michael. As talkative as ever, Michael was wrapping up his last year of A-level classes when I returned in 2007. He was having severe problems with his eyes, including bouts of momentary blindness, but his parents did not have the means to take him to a doctor to find out what was wrong. In addition, Margaret had lost her glasses and was trying to read by borrowing her husband's spectacles, which had a different prescription strength. She suffered constant headaches as a result. I found out that Mengo Hospital had an inexpensive eye clinic and referred them to it. Michael's problems were resolved with a simple prescription for eye drops, and Margaret was able to get her own glasses for 50,000 UGX (30 USD). Her headaches ceased immediately.

Michael took his A-level exams in 2008. He passed well in two subjects but did not get the scores needed in the third to get into university. So he started a short diploma course in business management instead. One often hears young people in Uganda like Michael repeat a common mantra of entrepreneurialism that masks state retreat: "We have to be job makers, not job seekers." And yet their access to capital to start businesses is also limited by banks' high interest rates (International Labour Office 2012, 41). So while Michael and other young people like him would like to exercise their entrepreneurial spirit, they often cannot.

Childhood Adversity—Beyond Orphanhood

The youth research assistants' own examples show that although orphanhood poses certain challenges, it does not tell the whole story of childhood adversity in Uganda. The juxtaposition of their situations attests to some of the issues that children, orphans and nonorphans alike, face on a daily basis. Though the scholarship on AIDS orphanhood has established certain patterns, these stories demonstrate that orphanhood intersects with many other factors to affect individual and family circumstances in a variety of ways. For many, it was not orphanhood itself but its potential consequence—poverty—that they felt most acutely as they grew up. These stories may therefore point to the longitudinal effects of misdirected interventions, such as those explained in part 1, that target orphanhood itself over poverty. The burden of orphanhood can be higher on girls like Sumayiya due to gendered experiences of orphanhood—from being forced out of her aunt's house to being forced out of school due to pregnancy—as well as a lack of extended-family and institutional support. Aside from herself, she also had to care for a younger sibling and a baby. Despite my assistance, her persistent poverty drove her to find whatever means she could to survive. However, she had different (and more lucrative if more risky) options than James, who also went to work to support himself and his family—and who also lost out on certain educational opportunities because of it. But despite these obstacles, both seem to have found their way and are doing better now than might have been predicted. By contrast, Malik benefited from having steady family support, but he and his family also struggled, and this struggle led his uncle to make choices that could easily have jeopardized Malik's access to educational opportunities. Malik had the most stable upbringing of the youth research assistants who lost parents, but this may also account for his prolonged dependence on his extended family.

Though his uncle's actions threatened to destabilize his education, his musical talent helped him get through school. But in the end, he has taken the longest to establish his own career and household.

Even with parents, the Obonyos have struggled to keep their children in school and might not have made it without outside support. Without it, Jill would not have reached university, but even a university education is not a promise of gainful employment. The Obonyos' story thus illustrates that this is an issue that affects youth and households more broadly, beyond the confines of orphanhood or even HIV/AIDS. Although I designed this project with youth research participation because I felt their experiences qualified the youth research assistants to study orphanhood, part of the impetus was admittedly also to give them some work skills and experience. Their ethnographic research with the younger cohort of the post-ARV generation thus helps us consider the ways AIDS orphanhood interacts with still other social factors to impact children and families, to be discussed in more detail in the next chapter.

6

Suffering, Silence, and Status: The Lived Experience of Orphanhood

[My brother] just comforts me and tells me not to worry; that everything will be fine. Other times we all just keep quiet and forget all our problems.

F A R Z A N A , a seventeen-year-old Ugandan girl who had taken care of four siblings
since the death of their parents when she was eleven years old (see appendix)

Silence too is a legitimate discourse on pain—if it is acknowledged.
F I O N A   R O S S (2001, 272)

The stories of young people in chapter 5 demonstrate some of the daily struggles that are common among young Ugandans—and young people throughout sub-Saharan Africa. AIDS is too often the subtext; a constant intermediary in African children's lives. Here, I draw heavily on the youth participatory research performed by the youth research assistants (RAs) with the younger cohort of the post-ARV (antiretroviral) generation who were born around the time antiretroviral therapy (ART) became more widely available in the early years of the twenty-first century. By doing so, I aim to provide a deeper understanding of the ways that children affected by AIDS actually experience orphanhood and explore the social context of AIDS as a both a cause of social suffering and a context for the suffering of individual children. As youth RA Sumayiya reflected—on both her own experiences and those of the children in her focus group—"HIV/AIDS has taken away the happiness of the young people, by making them become orphans; by taking away their rights to parental love; by taking away the right to education. It has led the young to suffering . . . since their parents are no more." Those who have lost parents or siblings to the disease are also affected by the illness and death of other adult interlocutors such as relatives and teachers, and not least of all their own risks of being infected. While many studies have acknowledged this to some extent, Arthur Kleinman and his coeditors suggest that "the relationship of suffering to meaning-making must be worked through if interventions (academic and practical) are to be adequate to the complexity of human problems and not romanticize or trivialize human conditions" (Kleinman, Das, and Lock 1997, xvi). It is thus important for us to understand how children feel about and deal with these circumstances. Three crucial concepts emerge from this analysis: suffering, silence, and status.

The word *suffering* has several meanings, most of them passive and not of the making of the one who experiences it: the dictionary lists various meanings for the root word *suffer*, such as "to undergo or feel pain or distress"; "to sustain injury, disadvantage, or loss"; "to undergo a penalty, as of death"; "to endure pain, disability, death, etc., patiently or willingly."[1] It is striking that AIDS thrusts all these experiences onto people, including children. Only the last definition implies a choice, but a constrained one at that—to endure; and this is what many children do, patiently and willingly, as they experience the passing of people close to themselves and sometimes succumb to AIDS themselves.

Much of this suffering, I argue, is exacerbated by people's penchant for silence about such suffering. Many adults discourage open dialogue with children over the reasons for—and sometimes even the fact of—their parents' deaths, thinking that it protects children from trauma. I initially found this avoidance of discussion deeply problematic, but my thinking about it evolved over the course of this study. The persistent silence surrounding HIV/AIDS can compound children's emotional suffering—even as increased poverty and family instability deepen their material suffering—but I also came to see that silence has some important social and protective uses, especially amid continued stigma. Approaching silence as a distinct form of communication rather than an absence of it (following Rogers et al. 1999), I consider silence's functions, its detriments and its consolations, in the context of HIV/AIDS–affected children's lives.

Much of this silence about suffering is in turn due to the continued stigma of HIV/AIDS in Uganda that makes one's status unspeakable—despite the adverse effect this silence has on the social order and efforts to eliminate the disease. After a brief discussion of the methodological challenges posed by such silences, I also give particular attention to children's and their caregivers' efforts to cope with their circumstances and secure the resources necessary for survival in the aftermath of parental loss. I end with a summary discussion of youth RAs' recommendations for appropriate responses to AIDS-affected children's suffering, including the contentious question of disclosure of HIV status.

Suffering and Its Antecedents

One way to think about what it means to suffer is to place suffering in its cultural context. Individual suffering cannot be properly understood without also understanding it in the context of broader social suffering, particularly in the midst of a widespread pandemic. There are significant continuities and departures of orphans' experiences in the age of HIV/AIDS that impinge on their feelings of suffering. Many informants—from policy makers to nongovernmental organization (NGO) workers to grandparents raising orphans to the children themselves—considered orphanhood at the hands of the AIDS virus to be much more traumatic than other means of becoming orphaned, including war. Baker Waiswa of Uganda Women's Effort to Save Orphans (UWESO) once told me, "Psychologically, the trauma of HIV-orphaned children is worse. It's multidimensional. . . . These ones have lost their parents, but they themselves could be HIV-positive. So . . . the psychological fear they have . . . in my opinion is worse than the war orphans. . . . These have seen their parents die of HIV/AIDS, but they too are afraid they could die of the same, and you know, it's a slow process depending on the infection they get."[2]

The extent of psychological impact of orphanhood depends to some extent on the age at which children become orphaned (Webb 2005, 235). Children who lose their parents when they are very young may have little or no memory of them, and if they are well integrated into their current households rather than singled out as orphans, their parents' deaths tend to have fewer debilitating psychological and developmental effects, as with Robin (see his story in the appendix). Most will in fact refer to their guardians as "mother" and "father." By contrast, singling out a child as an orphan may impede his or her integration into the adoptive household (Webb 2005, 233), as occurred with several of the children with whom we worked (again, see the appendix for the children's profiles). This is why humanitarian interventions that directly target orphans can be so problematic.

Even before that point, however, the slow death of a parent suffering from AIDS is what spurs children's anxieties. One vivid example from our study comes to mind: twins Wasswa and Kato,[3] who, at ten years old when we met them, had been watching their father slowly waste away from AIDS complications for years. Their mother had known she was HIV-positive, but she told no one, even after becoming pregnant with the twins. She thought being HIV-positive would embarrass her and her family. She also avoided ARVs, believing rumors that she would only die more quickly if she took them.[4]

Wasswa, the firstborn, had a natural birth, but Kato was delivered by cesarean section. Wasswa was therefore infected with HIV while Kato was not.

Their mother died when the boys were two years old, and their aunt Rose—whom they call "Jaaja" (Grandma) just like everyone else—took them in. She could see that Wasswa was a sickly boy, so she had him tested for HIV. When the test came back positive, she managed to get him enrolled in an antiretroviral program.

When we met them in 2007, their father had been living positively with

AIDS but had been bedridden for several years. They all stayed at their aunt's house with a dozen other orphaned cousins. The twins constantly stood by their father's bedside, attending to his every need. They kept assuring us that their father would be fine: "He will not be leaving us as well," they would say, indirectly referencing their mother's death. Kato especially stayed close to his father, despite his aunt's efforts to get him to go out and play with his friends. In fact, he became protective of both his father and his brother; when Wasswa failed to take his medicine (sometimes on purpose), Kato would fetch it and ensure that Wasswa took each tablet. Kato really loved school and hoped to be a doctor one day, but the constant illnesses and worry about losing their father always provided distractions that kept either boy from doing very well in school.

Silence and Emotional Suffering

Notwithstanding a significant reduction in the social stigma that caused Wasswa and Kato's mother to stay silent about her HIV status and avoid seeking treatment, there is still a notable culture of silence and (even deliberate) misinformation when it comes to informing children about the disease. For example, the twins had not been told that their father had AIDS. People living with HIV/AIDS will tend not to reveal their status freely, preferring instead to attribute the inscription of suffering on their bodies to various secondary infections (Parsons 2012, 121). The twins were thus told that their father had kidney failure (one of his AIDS symptoms) and would be getting an operation soon. Indeed, Wasswa was not even told that he was HIV-positive, though he had been on ARV medications since he was a toddler. Instead, they told him that he took so many medications because he had a "brain illness." Two other children in the household were HIV-positive and on ART, but they were supplied with different reasons why they needed the medicine. Kato had suspicions that his father and his twin brother were also HIV-positive, but he was too afraid to ask anyone. Instead, Kato continued to build dreams for the future that included him, his brother, and their father. In August 2012, however, the boys' father died. The whole family seemed to understand that he died of AIDS—as other family members had before him—but, despite reduced stigma in Uganda, no one dared utter the fact aloud, a fact that increased stress among the children in the household in particular. Such instances reflect the early twentieth-century philosopher Georg Simmel's observation: "Secrecy secures, so to speak, the possibility of a second world alongside of the obvious world, and the latter is most strenuously affected by the former" (1906, 462). Put another way at the end of that century, Annie G. Rogers and her colleagues have written, "The tension between what is known and what lies beneath the surface of conscious knowing, or what is spoken and what is known but not spoken, produces a phenomenon of double meaning that is common in our lives. We experience this doubling in a variety of ways, including living with contradictions, 'being of two minds' about something, and the internal dialogues that accompany ambivalence. These dialogues may be less conscious but are nevertheless evident in children's thinking" (Rogers et al. 1999, 86–87). The twins' father passed away just as doctors were slowly revealing to Wasswa that he had the same incurable disease as his father. One can only imagine what this does for a boy who is realizing he has the same affliction from which he has spent his entire childhood watching his father slowly die.

It was typical for guardians to stay quiet about AIDS infection, and even relatives' AIDS-related deaths, often based both on their own discomfort with the topic and on the assumption that silence protects children from trauma (Bauman and Germann 2005, 105–6), that they are "unable to bear the burden of knowing" (Lowenthal et al. 2014, 148). On the other hand, Anthony Swift and Stan Maher note that, in the South African context, "Many adults do not concern themselves with the feelings of children. While this tradition is changing, the relationship between children and grandparents, traditionally circumscribed, is especially slow in changing. And the taboo of talking about death and AIDS offers no candid conversation towards a child whose parent has died" (2008, 39). I take up the issue of intergenerational relationships and their changing dynamics as the burden of orphan care shifts predominantly onto grandparents in part 4, but suffice it to say here that, similar to South Africa or the British "stiff upper lip," in Uganda, rather than acknowledge children's emotional pain and loss, adults tended to keep quiet and children were taught silence and stoicism—ostensibly because "it is not in our culture" to talk about one's emotional pain. During this study, however, we saw that this silence mainly compounds children's emotional suffering. Their participation in this study seemed to have given many children a safe space in which to voice their suffering, but this was not necessarily the case outside of confidential exchanges with the researchers. While shielding them from information about AIDS is ostensibly intended to protect them, it means that children cannot articulate their fears or accurately process information about the progress of the disease, even as increased poverty and family instability due to AIDS deepens their material suffering.

We saw this pattern often in how children and families dealt with death: guardians regularly presumed that it was best to protect children from exposure to death, but several instances pointed to the opposite conclusion, given children's expressed desires for closure. "Nobody told me when my father died," Joanna, an eight-year-old girl, told her youth RA. Once he gained rapport with her, she talked about her father at length, lamenting that while her guardians constantly reminded her that she was an orphan, no one seemed willing to talk to her about her father. "I don't even have a picture of him," she lamented. Though studies report that children's development of an understanding of death can vary from ages five to twelve, experience with death helps advance their understanding of it (M. Mahon 2011, 63). Since children in Uganda are frequently exposed—at least indirectly—to death, it would follow that they develop capacities to process it from early ages, obviating the need to shield them from it or deny children opportunities to express their grief.

Studies have shown that children as young as six can also understand the implications of HIV infection (Geiselhart, Gwebu, and Kruger 2008, 111). Some children in our study indicated the need not only for closure but for *dis*closure—about their parents' deaths, and also about their own situation, thus further challenging conventional wisdom about children's ability to deal with death and/or medical knowledge. Jaaja Hamidah's household is a case in point: I first met Jaaja Hamidah on a drizzly morning in 2007 at the home of a mutual acquaintance. Jaaja came with the four children in her charge when she heard that a researcher wanted to talk to area families caring for AIDS orphans.[5] Jaaja had a lot to say on that topic—to me, anyway.

But first, Hamidah brought her youngest grandchild, Justine, to see us. Justine was a seven-year-old girl suffering from AIDS. She was a frail girl who looked like a malnourished five-year-old. Her face was gaunt, and her skinny body floated in an adult man's jacket Jaaja had put on her to keep her warm. Her skin was dry and ashy. She greeted me listlessly, and when I took her hand, it was on fire with fever. On this rainy morning, she seemed extremely sick, but she had come to talk to the *mzungu* (white person), so we proceeded with a brief interview. I gave her a banana, and she gobbled it up. She spoke quietly and sadly, but she answered our questions fairly directly.

I asked Justine where she lived before coming to stay with her grandmother, and Justine told me with some detachment about her father. "John [her older brother] told me we lived with our father," she said. "Daddy was working in town, so he brought us to live with Jaaja. Then he shifted to another place called Kawanda, which is far away. Grandmother tells me he is a mechanic. Daddy never visits us at all, and mommy is dead. She died while I was still young so I did not cry or do anything. I have never seen her, but Jaaja told me she died and I saw where she was buried. I would like to live with my daddy at Kawanda."

It is not that her grandmother is bad to her, she explained; she would just like to live with her father as well. Even so, Justine brightened considerably when we talked about her grandmother, who took care of her, her brother, and two of her cousins—all of whom lived with her in a two-room apartment. Justine was not in school because she was often ill, so her *jaaja* would stay in bed with her and sing her songs and tell her stories. The three boys were also fond of her, bringing her scavenged snacks from school and coming up with new bedside antics to keep her entertained. Though none were told of her HIV status, all the boys seemed to understand that Justine was sick and fragile, so while they would constantly play with her, they would treat her gently. They sang and danced for her to try to make her laugh. She listed only one friend, as many of the neighbors did not allow their children to play with her; she herself had not been told of her HIV status, so she was not sure why. "I often suffer from fever," she said. "Fever" is a common euphemism adults use for AIDS when talking to children to explain their or another's condition without naming it, describing the symptom rather than the disease. "I don't like injections. However, I like swallowing tablets," she added bravely. She did not mind if other children teased her about not living with her parents, either. "I used to feel bad, but the fact that I have a grandmother who loves me makes me happy."

This was the first and last time we ever saw Justine. She was admitted to the hospital shortly afterward and died about a month later from AIDS-related pneumonia.

As with many older children, Justine's older brother, twelve-year-old John, likely knew his HIV-positive status even though it was never explicitly disclosed to him. He was a bright and funny child to whom people young and old took immediately. He too contracted HIV perinatally. His *jaaja* took him to the hospital to get his medications, though she had, at the doctors' recommendation, delayed revealing his actual condition to him. Several guardians told us that doctors had recommended against disclosing an HIV-positive child's status to him until he is older, but John was an inquisitive boy who had a lot of questions as to why he and Justine took so many drugs and why Justine fell sick so often. "I think he already knows," his grandmother whispered to us as John played just out of earshot. She continued:

> One time while playing outside my house, his friends told him not to run so fast for there were rusted iron sheets nearby. His friends told him, "If those rusted iron sheets cut you, you will get tetanus and die." John responded, "I know I'm already dead. I will be dying anytime soon." Of course I faced him and told him never to say such a thing for he was too young to die, but deep in my heart it crossed [my mind] that maybe he had figured out he was

HIV-positive due to the constant visits we make to [name of] Hospital and the drugs he takes.

Despite all this, John seemed optimistic about his future. His face brightened when I asked him about his plans for the future, and he had lots of dreams. He said he wanted to be a doctor, perhaps so he would be able to cure his sister and himself and save their own lives. But when Justine fell sick, John got nervous. While Justine was in the hospital, her cousins were allowed to see her, but her brother was not. Their grandmother thought it would be too distressful for him, so she kept him away. When Justine passed away after a few weeks, he had not had a chance to say good-bye to his sister.

John took Justine's death as a harbinger of things to come: at her burial—which he *was* allowed to attend—he fainted repeatedly, moaning, "I'm next, I'm next."

"Don't say that! Don't say that!" relatives entreated him gently to reassure him. But John's mantra turned out to be a self-fulfilling prophecy, for he too succumbed quickly to pneumonia and died just two months after his sister.

Full Disclosure

The consequences of HIV prevention trends for today's children and youth are troubling considering caregivers' continued hesitancy to fully disclose to children the reasons for their parents' deaths, and—in the case of many HIV-positive children who were infected through birth—their own HIV status.

Nearly 1.7 million HIV-positive adolescents ages ten to nineteen were estimated to be living in sub-Saharan Africa in 2013—many of whom do not know their status. Even when they do, their access to treatment is significantly lower than that of adults (23 percent versus 37 percent; UNICEF 2014). In Uganda, the percentage of ART-eligible adolescents ages fifteen to nineteen who are receiving ART is estimated to be slightly higher at 29 percent—but only 17 percent of the estimated total number of adolescents ages fifteen to nineteen living with HIV are currently in any kind of care (Uganda AIDS Commission 2014, 23).

Ugandan law states that children under twelve years old (John's age when he died) may not voluntarily submit themselves for HIV testing (Sloth-Nielsen and Mezmur 2008, 290). Yet Klaus Geiselhart, Thando Gwebu, and Fred Kruger, who have shown that children as young as six can process the implications of HIV infection, believe that "the frequent claim that the children are too young is mostly an excuse for not wanting to, or not knowing how to, communicate about HIV and AIDS" (Geiselhart, Gwebu, and Kruger 2008, 111).

Such may be the case, but these matters are not so simple for guardians who are often ill equipped on a number of counts—and even guardians were not allowed to request HIV testing for children in their care unless there were clinical indications that the child may in fact be infected and thus require medical care for his or her condition (Sloth-Nielsen and Mezmur 2008, 290). This policy was taken to the opposite extreme with the passage of the 2014 HIV/AIDS Prevention and Control law that *requires* parents to tell their children of their status.[6] There was vociferous backlash against the passage of the law by many human rights advocates who fear that the law, which criminalizes "willful and intentional" HIV transmission, only discourages more people from knowing their own and their children's statuses (Bernard 2014). Though testing is now free on demand and the average age of disclosure has been dropping steadily with the wider availability of treatment (World Health Organization 2011), none of the guardians in our study were encouraged to disclose status to HIV-positive children before twelve years of age. National guidelines permit health workers to disclose children's HIV status starting from twelve years old (Katabira et al. 2008, 4),[7] so guardians often leave it to medical professionals. But the doctors of the HIV-positive children in our study did not begin the gradual disclosure process until the children were well into their teens.

The disconnect between policy and practice reflects a more general societal hesitancy, even within the law and the medical community, to disclose HIV status. Anthropologist and psychotherapist Ross Parsons recalls an incident in Zimbabwe when even a doctor who had treated a pediatric AIDS patient throughout his childhood and adolescence suddenly "realized," upon preparing to transfer his patient to an adult clinic, that he and his patient had never actually discussed being HIV-positive. "I began to assume that he must know," the doctor shrugged (Parsons 2012, 111). Elizabeth Lowenthal and colleagues found similar challenges when rolling out a child disclosure support program in Botswana: "Early in the development of our model . . . healthcare workers tended to perceive disclosure as being the responsibility of family. At the same time, cultural practice in Botswana was to shield children from bad news (such as HIV status and even death of parents)" (Lowenthal et al. 2014, 18). This tendency is not limited to sub-Saharan Africa, either: parents in London tended to delay disclosure of their children's HIV diagnoses as well (Waugh 2003). However, as Jaaja Rose's family demonstrated, certain children like Wasswa may not *want* to be told—even when they may already "know" on some level. This consideration is difficult to weigh, though, against the experiences of children like John, who seemed to really want someone to level with him. That is why giving children the choice to be independently and confidentially informed is important. A number of clinical studies, most of them conducted before the reversal of HIV prevalence, have found no significant psychological effects of disclosure and have recommended full disclosure to adolescents (Bikaako-Kajura et al. 2006), but it would be interesting to see whether attitudes may have changed over a time when discussion of HIV/AIDS has supposedly become more open than in the past while at the same time subjected to moralizing policy discourses. The PEPFAR rollout of ARV (2004–7) may have commuted death sentences for many people living with HIV, but it has been replaced by other moralizing discourses, such as abstinence-only sex education, that effectively make HIV infection a "choice" by blaming the victim. Such discourses continue to hinder the creation of more openness around HIV status and treatment.

It is also crucial to consult children and young people on their opinions about when and how to disclose the status of HIV-positive children to them. More child- and youth-centered social action research on the issue of disclosure and HIV/AIDS–related policies is thus urgently needed, research that also takes into account issues of intergenerational dependence.

Hearing the younger children's stories gave occasion for the youth RAs to reflect on their own experiences of orphanhood—thereby providing a retrospective view of their emotional needs as orphaned children as well as a longitudinal understanding of the effects of nondisclosure of their parents' HIV status on children. The silences around the youth RAs' parents' deaths continued to haunt them into adolescence and adulthood. In a debriefing interview with me six months into the project, Malik, a twenty-year-old youth RA at the time, recalled the last time he saw his mother:

> I saw my mum when she was dying though I didn't figure out then that she was dying. But I remember my grandmother ordered us to get out of the house at that instant and then when I reached outside and peeped back, I could see my grandmother covering my mother with a white piece of cloth. I was seven years old . . . I was staying with my [maternal] uncle. My mum had given him money and told him to take care of me and ensure that I went to school (which he didn't do), but later when my mother was on her deathbed, I was brought to her. I spent one night and next morning I was told to come sit beside her and wipe her face. After wiping it I realized something was wrong and it was then that I was sent out and a white cloth covered over her face.
>
> They didn't want me to know what was going on. I had never seen my granny do that so there and then I knew something was wrong. Later my other

granny came and explained that mum was dead, and we should stay calm. However, I wasn't calm. It was hard!

My fears there and then were that I couldn't live without my mum, so I just didn't know what my life was going to become. I loved my mum so much, you know . . .

I was young, so I don't even know what my mum died of; no one talks about it, and I am afraid of bringing it up even now. I was scared at that time, I had no idea that she was going to die, and I took long to believe she died; even up to now I don't believe it.

Because no one had explained what was going on to him, Malik was—and to some degree continues to be—bewildered by his mother's death. Margaret Mahon points out that "acknowledging the reality of an impending death provides an extremely important opportunity within families. A child saying good-bye to a dying parent is exceedingly difficult, but can be very beneficial for the child" (Mahon 2011, 81). Even at the funeral, it is not too late to provide children with opportunities to say good-bye, but this did not seem to be happening with children we spoke with in Uganda; even as children like Malik grow up and gain some distance from the event, they continue to fear raising the subject with relatives, who also preferred to linger at the edge of conscious knowing rather than speak the unspeakable (Rogers et al. 1999).

In *Mourning and Melancholia*, Sigmund Freud described the psychological tasks involved in mourning as "the acceptance of loss, the introjection of important facets of that which is lost and then the 'letting go' of the lost" (1917, as cited in Parsons 2005, 76). It seems that this process is sometimes thwarted by the curtailing of discussion with children about death.

Youth RA James had lost his father, who died suddenly of a heart attack when James was twelve years old. In one conversation, he compared his experiences with Jaaja Hamidah's family, whom he visited during the study. He saw it this way:

The other boys [cousins] don't really understand what John and Justine died of; however, they fear hospitals now—and falling sick. They kind of don't understand what's going on and the adults around them can't give those answers.

When my father died, people didn't talk to me or explain what was going on; however, they would come tell me stories to try to make me forget and not think about it. I didn't instantly forget but it kind of helped me. . . . The adults around me didn't really explain except I heard my mother explain to my brother and other people. I never asked her then but after some time I asked my brother and he explained that my dad had died of high blood pressure. There is some kind of separation, as in adults don't want to talk about it to the children, yet actually the children talk about it amongst themselves and ask lots of whys.

In this case, the other boys are really worried because they don't understand why their cousins are dead, so they are confused, thinking they might die soon too, and no one is coming out to give them the right answers.

Silence and Its Consolations

People living with HIV/AIDS often purport to want to protect their children, and they see such silences and misdirection as meeting their responsibilities to do so. Even the fact of orphanhood is often played down, as evidenced by the selective use of vernacular terms such as the Luganda *balekwa* for "orphans."[8] Guardians agreed that orphans suffer more today than when they are growing up because it is harder to provide for them and integrate them into the extended family, which is fragmenting under the constraints of daily life under HIV/AIDS and poverty (as will be explored further in chapter 7). Yet younger children especially did not know much about the previously discussed term *mulekwa* ("orphan"), and even when they did, few identified with it.

With the increasing availability of pediatric ARV treatment, HIV-positive children have become both emblematic of success in the fight against AIDS and a threat to it in that they may survive to infect others with HIV. This dual role also has implications for the questions of when to disclose their status to HIV-positive children. Caregivers maintain certain silences regarding the children in their care in a context of extreme stigma; despite Uganda's reputation for success in battling HIV infection and the availability of antiretroviral medication, the social stigma associated with the disease is still strong and has in fact taken on new forms. The knowledge that someone was taking medication could be interpreted as an expression of admiration for the person's recovery from HIV/AIDS symptoms, but it could also reflect a fear that ARVs hid the visible signs of HIV/AIDS in one's social circles (Seeley 2014, 100–101). In this regard, silence and concealment constitute an act of protection, respect, and honor—one that is always embodied and relational (Hardon and Posel 2012; Moyer 2012, S76). As the twins' aunt aptly put it, "So many people take ARVs; however, you will never hear of anyone dying of AIDS." I would add that you also rarely hear of anyone *living* with AIDS—but you certainly see them. She continued:

> Even with all the ARVs, sensitization, mobilization, etc., people still look at AIDS as this "big curse" or "disease of sin." . . . Some people in rural areas still associate AIDS with witchcraft, so in brief, some homes and communities still victimize AIDS patients, in a big home like mine where I have so many young

children all with different parents and different characters. On a bad day while playing, they might fight as kids and insult each other, so imagine a situation where one of them goes like, "No wonder you have this bad disease, AIDS, and will die soon!" It would definitely hurt the HIV-positive child.

Given the social consequences of others knowing one's HIV status, people are still unlikely to reveal it to others. Children orphaned by AIDS, and particularly HIV-positive children, can easily be ostracized by adults, both within and outside their households. Children known or suspected of being HIV-positive are often physically and socially isolated by the community. Wasswa's aunt told us, "In some families and communities, the adults make the HIV-positive kids feel really different from the other kids. They have special cups and plates for them; they are not allowed to play with the other children. . . . However, it is not the case here, so maybe that's what delayed Wasswa's knowing his HIV status." In the context of continued stigma, then, the family's silence and concealment of HIV status engendered a sense of normalcy for the HIV-positive children in the household by not singling them out for special treatment.

In any case, silence definitely has its uses. Similarly, silence around AIDS as an agent of parents' deaths may be justified as a means of preserving memories of the deceased against the stigma of AIDS—a stigma that can indeed tarnish them even in death.

From a public health perspective, maintaining silence still seems deeply problematic, especially as children get older and become sexually active, since children are not always well informed about HIV transmission and prevention (Geiselhart, Gwebu, and Kruger 2008, 107). These good intentions, then, could well have extensive adverse consequences for children and the community; underestimating their capacity to understand and cope with HIV/AIDS–related information can not only deepen children's bewilderment at a loved one's decline and death but also expose them to greater risk of HIV infection (and infection of others if they are already infected). On the other hand, we heard many stories about children taking the news very badly and starting to behave recklessly. For example, Wasswa's aunt told us, "I have seen households where, once a child gets to know they have AIDS, they deliberately decide to spread it to the others who are not their biological siblings with one sense in their head: 'Why do I have it and so-and-so doesn't have it?'" In fact, Wasswa began to act out after the death of his father. He was all right at school despite slipping grades, but he would lash out unexpectedly at people at home. He even stopped taking his ARVs until his brother Kato pleaded with him to take care of himself. "You're the only family I have left, so if you die, I'll be all alone," he reminded his twin. Wasswa agreed to go back on his ARV therapy, and his family, figuring he just needed to get away from the house—and indeed the very room—where his father had died, put the twins in the boarding section at school.

Initially, I had assumed that the purposeful concealment of HIV/AIDS status acted as a source of tension in families like Jaaja Rose's, but over time I came to see that perhaps in situations where young patients do not know their status, concealment actually prevents tension while preserving the dignity of the child. Things became so much tenser in the household when Wasswa came to know his status; he was angry, distrustful, and scared. Things turned out fine, but the episode made Rose even more wary of informing Travis, another HIV-positive child in her care who was doing extremely well in school at the time, that he too carried the same potential for disease; they did not want to throw him off his game.

Silence, then, has both its detriments and its advantages—and silence does not always equal secrecy but rather a pact that people honor for the sake of the other (Moyer 2012). Josien de Klerk has posited that "a core element within compassionate care is concealment. Concealment is not denial; nor is it completely explicable by theories of stigma. It is a 'core orientation'—a 'language' in a society focused on enclosure, trust and social position. Concealment is ingrained in everyday practice" (de Klerk 2012, S36). While concealment of HIV status is not without its consequences, we as a research team also became more appreciative of the reasons for it as we did the research, but respecting those silences also made it harder to know what children think about it. Despite the abundance of research on children's experiences with death in Western contexts, we need more research to understand AIDS orphanhood's psychosocial impact (Webb 2005, 235–37; M. Mahon 2011, 64) in Africa and elsewhere. But silence and concealment of children's statuses pose vexing methodological challenges.

Suffering, Silence, and Their Challenges for HIV/AIDS Research with Children

The silences around suffering in general and disclosure of children's HIV-positive status in particular are precisely what posed methodological and ethical challenges for us as child-centered researchers; for example, I was eager to talk to Wasswa and Kato about their feelings about their father's illness, as well as Wasswa's slow realization that he too was HIV-positive. He seemed to need to have someone acknowledge his fears and anxieties. Yet, we could not talk directly to them about it, because the family had never discussed the fact that their father had AIDS. Further, though adults in the family, teachers, and the research team all knew that Wasswa was HIV-positive, he did not know that we knew—and we were not even sure of the degree to which he himself knew, even on some intuitive level. And yet we knew, his aunt knew, his teachers knew, and even his brother at least sensed it. Though his aunt had told us and his teachers of his status, no one within the household acknowledged it to anyone else. But we as researchers were also bound by the silences that prevailed in the community. It was not our place to disclose to the children any of the information the family withheld, so we decided that we would wait and see whether any of the HIV-positive children with whom we were working would broach the subject with any of their youth RAs. If not, however, we would just have to let it rest. Silence, however, can also be analyzed as a form of language of the unsayable that constitutes a presence rather than an absence (Rogers et al. 1999), and we as researchers must thus attend to it.

Kleinman, Das, and Lock argue that "withholding acknowledgment of pain is a societal failure . . . the study of suffering, therefore, needs to interrogate this failure of theory" (1997, xvi). Considering the stakes in revealing HIV status amid continued stigma would seem to question this statement to some extent. Drawing on anthropological theories of human suffering, one can better examine the difficulties that accompany the loss of close kin to AIDS. "It is not in our culture" may be an insufficient explanation of why guardians maintain silence around HIV/AIDS-affected children, yet the continued stigma of HIV-positive status presents a compelling mitigating circumstance as a condition that remains unspeakable: though caregivers acknowledged that their silence was driven by stigma associated with AIDS and the desire to protect children, they also told us that they felt overwhelmed and inadequately prepared to discuss HIV status with children. Jaaja Rose once told us:

> The twins are in P.6 [sixth grade] now and at this stage, the schools begin teaching them about sex, STDs, the reproductive system and adolescence. On one day after they had a lesson about AIDS, [Wasswa] returned home sullen and sad. When I tried to engage him he mentioned they had studied about AIDS at school because the teachers wanted the children to know how to protect themselves against that killer disease. The look in his eyes clearly showed he had so many questions—questions that I couldn't answer. So I just let the issue drop when the child didn't say anything more; I got scared.

Such insecurities may force guardians into a silence of convenience, bolstered by medical experts who can mediate and a set of cultural prohibitions on conversations of a certain nature between generations. Many caregivers' default position is therefore just to wait and let the children figure it out over time. As with Malik having to guess to this day exactly what caused his mother's death, many caregivers of HIV-positive children wait to see whether the child's status will eventually just dawn on them as they learn more about HIV/AIDS and match the proposed care regiments to their own. However, adults' reluctance to disclose such information to children is fueled by the impulse to protect children from their circumstances, rather than ameliorating them. So while nondisclosure may be understandable on one level, we have to consider the long-term implications of these decisions for children—however difficult it is to engage in such research.

In her groundbreaking study with terminal pediatric cancer patients in the United States, Myra Bluebond-Langner (1978) discovered children's awareness of impending death—despite mutual pretense between children and parents that the child would survive—not by directly questioning children but by overhearing what they said to other children on the ward (similar to how Jaaja Hamidah discovered that John knew something of his own condition by overhearing him) and also by noting indicative behavior such as giving away toys. Mahon cautions, however, that we cannot presume too much about how children grieve, as their grief can be not only qualitatively different from that of adults but also cannot always be gauged just by observation—especially when children purposely conceal their feelings (M. Mahon 2011, 83).

Ethical questions also arise in the rush to analyze silence and suffering. In such difficult circumstances, researchers are also obligated to bear witness through empathetic listening, or what Parsons calls "to sit with affect": "Sitting with affect, for therapists, generally means tolerating painful feelings without glossing over them in pursuit of either 'solutions' or our own emotional comfort. A true account of suffering, one that acknowledges both destruction and resilience, requires attention too to that which is in danger of being hidden, either through being subsumed by other pressing realities or because it elicits from us fear and denial of emotional pain" (Parsons 2005, 77). Parsons notes that his work as an ethnographer of HIV-positive children in Zimbabwe leaves him more personally exposed to others' grief than as a therapist, where self-protection measures are built into the disciplinary methodology. But perhaps this kind of patient empathy is what it takes to draw out children who are not used to expressing their grief—and such cultural taboos might actually make it easier for children to express their grief to a researcher from outside their immediate community. I was not able to achieve this willingness of expression with children until they were older and had gained some distance from events, however; the youth RAs were more willing and able to articulate their grief at the loss of their parents than the young children in our study were, but some young children were also willing to confide in the youth RAs—another benefit of having youth RAs closer to them in age interact with them in data collection.

Children's Strategies for Dealing with Suffering

> In common sense as in scientific discourse, to survive means—one supposes—to undergo suffering. Both terms are important: "to undergo" implies passivity; "suffering" has a negative connotation. In this sense, surviving is a passion. Breaking with this approach consists on the contrary in saying that "survival is not only what remains, it is living the most intensely."
>
> DIDIER FASSIN (2007b, 261–62)

Efforts to understand children's suffering at the hands of orphanhood must be rooted in the present context of the African AIDS pandemic. Ahistorical analyses will fail to reveal suffering's true nature (Farmer [1992] 2006, 256). Those trying to understand children's experiences in difficult circumstances typically make this mistake by assuming that childhood itself is ahistorical and apolitical. When the AIDS pandemic still so seriously threatens children's survival, they too must participate in ameliorating the painful consequences for themselves, often by employing creative survival and coping strategies. By giving particular attention to children's efforts—independent of their caregivers—to secure the resources necessary for survival in the aftermath of parental loss, we may gain a better understanding of the needs that children themselves prioritize—and the ways in which they do indeed "live most intensely."

From a young age, children tend to seek resources at the local level through identification of broader social networks most likely to render assistance. For example, the youth RAs observed that children often made friends with peers who were better off than they were but who were also generous and willing to share their bounty. A first-grade girl in our study told us how she loved her "best friend" because she had given her an old pair of shoes, and she always shared the snacks she brought to school. In this way, she was able to leverage her vulnerability by raising the social status of another child who showed her generosity. The maintenance of the "best friend" title encouraged the friend's continued generosity toward her. Building support networks with other children may thus be one of the main advantages children see of going to school. It also provides some routine and regularity, as well as the possibility of getting an education itself that might alleviate the suffering of poverty.

Others may utilize broader community networks. Edwin, a clever nine-year-old boy, spent most weekends roaming the neighborhood in search of local celebrations, from birthdays to funerals. He had even ranked which families tended to have the best food at their gatherings so he could make the rounds and get fed by charming his neighbors. Few chased him away, knowing that his elderly grandmother cared for thirteen more grandchildren in a dilapidated brick house with a dirt floor, no windows, and little food. Some children may actually try to cultivate kin-like relationships with unrelated but well-meaning adults (including anthropologists) to try to supplement the limited support they get from their de facto caregivers—a strategy on which I elaborate in the next section.

Maureen Kendrick and Doris Kakuru talk of "funds of knowledge" of orphaned Ugandan children (particularly those in child-headed households) as a way of advancing "the view of children as resourceful, competent, and knowledgeable, highlighting their ability to build on, utilize, and acquire new funds of knowledge while simultaneously recognizing their conditions of extreme adversity" (2012, 398). Though some children in our study group found more social and/or material stability and resources over the course of the study by expanding their knowledge base or shifting to other households within their kin groups, it seemed many of them were still living hand to mouth or experiencing hardships several years into the study. These recurrent setbacks made it difficult for them to get beyond the point of bare survival.

As for emotional coping, children employed imaginative strategies. Many of the children in our study responded to anxiety about their circumstances by imagining stability, even where it could not be found. For example, as Wasswa and Kato witnessed the slow decline of their father's health, they continued to rationalize that "Daddy can't leave us," figuring that as their only surviving parent, he would have to hang on. Unfortunately, though, cultivating this idea did not help them to cope with his eventual death.

As they got older, the children started to engage in more active remembrance of lost loved ones and talk more openly about their parents. Robin, who could not remember anything about his father who died when he was an infant, started telling his youth RA in some detail about him. It only helped that people in his household—including the mother and siblings of his late father—were receptive to his questions, helping him fill in details in his story of his father's life. Robin's experience contrasts sharply with Joanna's longing for information about her father or James's earlier account of his father's death, when people would try to comfort him by distracting him and encouraging him to forget, rather than remember, his father. Children will find ways to express awareness of their parents' deaths and process the event. Norah's family did not like to talk about her deceased parents, though we learned from the picture of her household that she drew for us that they were buried

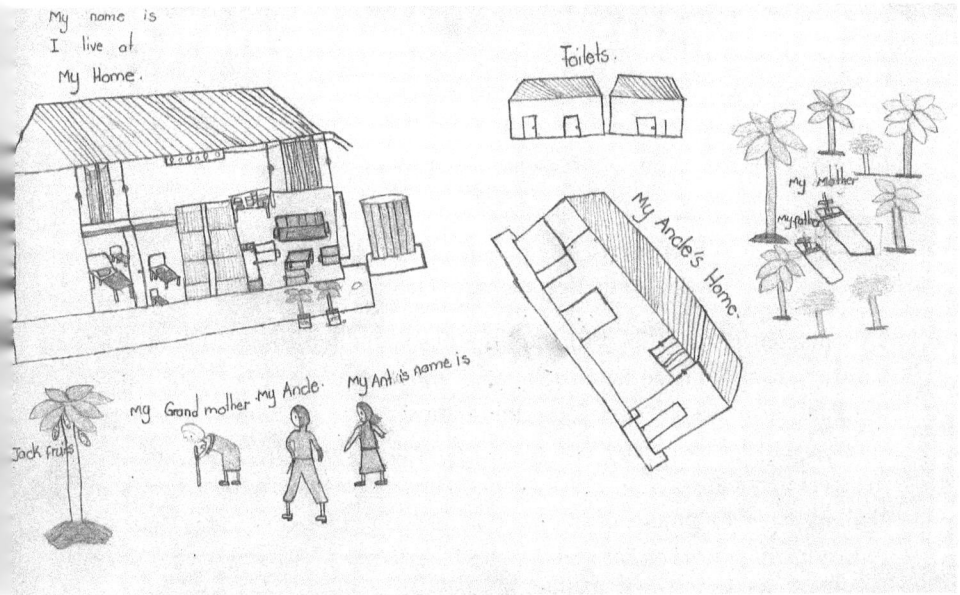

FIGURE 9. Norah, a double orphan, provided this drawing of her homestead, with her parents' graves in the upper right corner.

in the banana grove (fig. 9). Whereas the graves were not prominent or central in her picture, it was clear from her inclusion of them that her parents still had a presence in her life. By drawing the graves, she also prompted us to ask about them and then was able to discuss her parents' deaths and what she remembered about them.

Some children may not find many positive outlets for their grief and frustration, however: Zack, a teenager when we met him and his four siblings living on their own, was certainly bitter toward the extended family that abandoned him and his siblings after both their parents died (see the appendix for a more detailed description of Farzana's household). He was the most sullen and distrustful of his siblings. One uncle who lived nearby occasionally paid school fees for the older children, including Zack, whenever he could, but there were repeated delays in Zack's education, and when he did go to school, he did not perform well. At sixteen, he was still trying to complete the third grade, but his reports were dismal. The fact that he was so much older than the other children earned him the nickname *jaaja* (grandfather)—a nickname he did not embrace. He lashed out at whoever teased him, causing even more problems for him at school. However, he went on to finish his primary education and in 2013, he trained to be a mechanic.

Other children opened up to the study team about their current hardships, but it became apparent that they still had some resilience. Youth RA Michael described Jessie from his study group: "After some time she told me, 'Oh, grandmother kind of mistreats me,'—that kind of thing, you know? But, when you look at her, she's the type of person who has, she has *hope*, you know, she has hope and she sees something good."

"From Hard Life to Soft Life": Formulating Appropriate Responses to Orphan Suffering

This chapter has described some of the lived experiences of AIDS orphanhood as a constant negotiation with death and an intermediary in daily family life. Paul Farmer asserts that "describing suffering, no matter how touchingly, is not a sufficient scholarly response to the explanatory challenges posed by the world pandemic of HIV disease. . . . Perspectives for the near future are all illuminated by a mode of analysis that links the ethnographically observed to historically given social and economic structures" (Farmer [1992] 2006, 253). Farmer's point raises the broader issue of widespread poverty and how orphaned children's experience may or may not differ from that of other children. Previous studies have demonstrated that orphanhood makes little difference in communities suffering disproportionately from poverty and HIV (Joint Learning Initiative on Children and HIV/AIDS 2009, 3). However, this finding does not speak to children's psychosocial needs in the context of AIDS-related death; while it is true we must be careful not to reify orphans or AIDS orphanhood, we must also be careful not to presume that "they're just like other children," especially when it comes to their emotional needs. This presumption means something very different for foreign and local policy makers as well as adults and children.

In our final youth RA workshop in 2009, the research team characterized these challenges and agreed that there was a need to keep chipping away at HIV/AIDS stigma—and not reinforcing differential treatment of orphans by singling them out for aid. Then the conversation turned to appropriate responses to the identified needs—to which they gave some rather surprising responses that may in fact have been a response to conducting a study on orphanhood with a Western researcher. The youth RAs argued that conventional Western psychological models do not easily apply here; the context of children's everyday realities in Africa is hard, and how childhood is constructed in a given environment—for example, in which children sometimes receiving physical discipline is seen as formative—really matters for how the fact of their orphanhood should influence the behavior of adults toward them. The youth RAs agreed that it would be disadvantageous to treat orphans solely with kid gloves, but precautions still needed to be taken. Faridah felt conflicted over the imperative to treat orphans the "soft" way versus conventional wisdom about child discipline in which "you really just have to be hard on them. . . . So I'm wondering, are these two things competing?" A heated debate ensued:

JILL: No, okay, look, remember that they're already hard kids, they're hard-[ened] by their situation, they're already orphans, yeah? And if you beat them, remember they already have something, like, "People are not going to upset me." . . . because if this is your kid and you beat her, she's like, "Mommy has beaten me, what," but the [orphan], she's already hard, she lost her mom. If you beat her, she's not going to take it normal, like the way you're going to beat your kid. She'll take it like . . . "It's because my mom is not here." You inflict more pain! But if you talk to them, they'll feel like, "Oh, he couldn't even beat me," I mean, he'll feel like . . .

MICHAEL: You shouldn't make the kid understand that she'll jump from hard life to soft life [by being orphaned]. You should take it slowly. You should let the kid know that sometimes, these things are supposed to happen in order to get you somewhere.

FARIDAH: We have to understand that these are African children we are dealing with.

MICHAEL: You're right.

KRISTEN: So, you're saying you also need to continue to be firm, not necessarily beating them, but you still need to be firm . . .

JILL: . . . a person who is being caned by a father and mother will appreciate it, yeah, "It's the person who gave birth to me." But, a person who is being caned by a teacher or someone else will take it seriously that, "I'm being hated."

Although the youth RAs could not quite agree on disciplinary approaches, they did concur that integration in and strengthening of the family were important ways to improve the circumstances of the orphaned children with whom they conducted two years of fieldwork—but again, this did not mean entirely foregoing discipline and creating a "soft life" for a child whose social realities are in fact "hard."

This discussion must be placed in the context of ongoing debates in Uganda about corporal punishment. Although the law has prohibited corporal punishment in schools since 1998, this rule has rarely been enforced due to widespread endorsement of corporal punishment as an appropriate disciplinary measure for children. Nevertheless, children's rights activists tried to strengthen opposition to corporal punishment by including an article that would ban *all* corporal punishment in the Children Act amendments proposed to Parliament in 2015. However, the article could not garner enough popular support, so the provision was withdrawn from the bill, which eventually gained approval from Parliament in March 2016 with an article that instead strengthens the prohibition of corporal punishment in schools (Global Initiative to End All Corporal Punishment of Children 2016). The amendments were signed by the president and passed into law in May 2016.

The stories related in this chapter thus illustrate that children's understandings of AIDS as an agent of life and death are complex. They are marked by unwitting and willful ignorance, wishful denial, and silent acquiescence. The Ugandan government has been praised for its handling of the HIV/AIDS epidemic, but stigma still prevails—and in fact has been rejuvenated by Uganda's success at reducing its prevalence and making ARVs widely available (Whyte 2014). Lack of information—on their parents' or their own health—is meant to protect orphans from the harsh realities of illness and death, but it often means that children are left to process these experiences on their own, without guidance. Recognizing this situation, the task is to define which differences between orphans and nonorphans matter most to children, and exactly how. Given children's varied individual responses to difficult circumstances, it may not be appropriate to generalize. But this is no reason not to try to better discern patterns and best practices appropriate to the context. Silence has its social function, but children desired some acknowledgment of loss.

Perhaps the best place to start, then, is to cautiously break the silences around orphan suffering. As the stigma around AIDS gradually lessens, perhaps being an orphan or even an HIV-positive child will not be so "abnormal" that it must be kept secret, and children can feel both supported and protected.

PART FOUR

Blood Binds: The Transformation of Kinship and the Politics of Adoption

Orphanhood and the Transformation of Kinship, Fosterage, and Children's Circulation Strategies

Part 4 gradually returns to a broader political economy of orphanhood by considering the ways AIDS orphanhood and its attendant responses, from individual families and local African communities to the international community, have generated some significant effects. In this chapter, I examine the way AIDS orphanhood has influenced child circulation and kin construction in Uganda. While many studies have documented the effects of AIDS on orphans and vulnerable children's circulation in Africa (e.g., Nyambedha and Aagaard-Hansen 2003), few studies have critically examined the effects of AIDS on constructions of kinship, and particularly the role of "blood as a bodily substance of everyday significance with a peculiarly extensive symbolic repertoire" (Carsten 2011, 19). While "blood" in the African context has gained notoriety in the age of HIV/AIDS as a substance that carries pathogens such as the human immunodeficiency virus, it has also gained significance as a substance that immutably binds children orphaned by those pathogens to their extended kin, on whom they rely for care. Here, I trace the sometimes contradictory social, economic, and emotional effects of children's circulation within and across family networks, highlighting orphaned children's concerns with intrafamily mobility. By doing so, I show how orphan care in the age of HIV/AIDS is consequently transforming both fosterage practices and kin obligation, jeopardizing children's well-being and their ability to identify with the "blood ties" that still form powerful tropes of relatedness for them.

Despite the continued importance of "blood" as an idiom of relatedness and "home" as a place tied to the patrilineage, the presence of paternal kin in Ugandan orphaned children's lives is waning as more paternal family members relinquish their traditional obligations to absorb orphans, leaving the responsibility to maternal kin. Yet paternal kin continue to play an important symbolic role in the imaginations of Ugandan children, who still "belong" to their paternal clans by virtue of their shared "blood." Even while social ties with paternal kin wane, creating many adverse material and emotional effects for orphaned children, the concept of shared blood and the paternal "home" gains poignant significance for orphans in danger of becoming "rootless."

Fostering and Child Circulation in Africa: The Literature

Anthropologists have long been interested in Africa's enduring tradition of child circulation within extended kin networks and communities, much of which is applicable in the Ugandan context. Classic anthropological analyses of the circulation of children throughout Africa, such as those of Esther and Jack Goody (Goody and Goody 1969) tied the spatial movement of children to various social constructions of kinship. Whether they analyzed the circulation of children within the framework of structural-functionalism or understood the phenomenon as part of society-wide or individual adaptive strategies, anthropologists typically tried to understand the circulation of children within the "cultural logic" of the societies within which it took place. Summarizing the literature on African fostering practices, Sangeetha Madhavan points out that "child fostering provides an opportunity for both natal and fostering households to strengthen social and kinship ties through short- and long-term benefits to both parties, including reciprocity obligations, social security, access to resources (e.g., land), and investments in both households by sharing the costs of child rearing" (2004, 1444). Foster parents of children may not necessarily be related, but Catrien Notermans has observed that "system-oriented approaches to fosterage and kinship tend to adopt cultural ideals and to emphasize bonds of solidarity, mutual help and harmony in the African family" (2008, 357). Looking at dynamics at the household level, however, and at the ways children understand and experience the everyday dynamics of fostering reveals a different story, of tensions and contradictions in the motivations for fostering. Indeed, Caroline Bledsoe and Uche Isiugo-Abanihe wrote in 1989 that "many people provide support for children because children are useful to invest in, rather than simply because they must be supported somehow" (443). Often, fostering binds children and their caregivers in relationships of reciprocity or "paying it forward," or sometimes both. This bind is important for thinking about how fostering has evolved to the present day under the strain of structural factors such as the AIDS pandemic and deepening poverty.

Anthropological studies of fosterage and kinship in general declined in the 1980s, partly due to the dissolution of the discrete domains of economics, politics, religion, and kinship that had defined anthropology (Carsten 2000, 13). In the 1990s, demographers picked up the anthropological interest in fosterage, but with an economic cost-benefit analysis of the practice that Notermans argues "has to do with a rhetoric of dichotomies that typifies the demographic debates: the dichotomy between traditional and modern society, between rural and urban society, and between kinship structures and a cash economy" (2004, 48). Development organizations entered the fosterage debate in the first decade of the twenty-first century through the lens of aid to orphans and vulnerable children (OVC). This involvement led to interventions that at first treated OVC as an aid target—reifying them from kin networks—and then refocused on extended-family networks by building their capacity to absorb a growing number of orphans (see chapter 2). Despite some attention to extended-kin networks' coping mechanisms, the field of development studies has called for reinforcement of idealized traditional kin formations rather than identifying the tensions and transformations under way. While "kinship has to be brought back into anthropological theory on fosterage" (Notermans 2004, 48), it should also be better understood within development studies. Relatedly, children's studies scholars have criticized development practitioners for paying even less attention to children's choices and expressed interests than kinship in care provisioning.

How Orphanhood is Changing Kin and Care Dynamics: From "Voluntary" to "Crisis" Fostering

Fostering children has always to some extent been based on mutual interests under resource constraints. In her 1980s fieldwork on Mende grandmothers who foster young children, Bledsoe listed numerous motivations (economic, educational, emotional, and ritual) for parents, children, and proxy caregivers such as "grannies" in the circulation of children. She and Isiugo-Abanihe together asserted, "Minding a child is one of the most potent levers a granny can gain over the limited resources of a young cash earner, even if it is her own child" (1989, 465). But these characteristics generally applied to voluntary fostering. Development studies scholars have noted qualitative changes to OVC care that necessitate intervention. Aspaas (1999) and Oleke, Blystad, and Rekdal (2005) talk of "crisis fostering" in Africa in the context of AIDS, but whether the proliferation of orphans due to AIDS constitutes a 'crisis' is heavily debated. Esther Goody noted that among the Gonja of Ghana, fostering orphans "is a normative social obligation rather than a politically or economically motivated rationale" that drives purposive fostering (1982, 33). However, development practitioners argue that this obligation is being taxed

by the heavy social and economic effects of AIDS; reciprocal obligations become less important in such circumstances, especially when the biological
parent of a fostered child dies and thus cannot reciprocate. Though the people who foster their deceased relatives' children may not necessarily see it
as "crisis fostering" (Madhavan 2004, 1450), the circumstances under which
fosterage occurs today are nonetheless seen by communities and caregivers as
more traumatic, prompted by crisis in the form of death, as opposed to, say,
choices such as the pursuit of education. Decisions about who cares for children after their caregivers have died typically take place at the caregiver's funeral—overwhelmingly without the consultation of the children concerned
but often with considerations about which relatives have the time and money
to care for children predominating.[1]

Tatek Abebe and Asbjorn Aase critique the static distinctions drawn by
researchers and practitioners between "rupturing, transient, adaptive, and
capable families," pointing out that they are in fact part of a continuum along
various dimensions of orphan care (2007, 2062). Labeling AIDS orphanhood
a "crisis" that makes OVC targets of aid obscures the plasticity and adapt-
ability of traditional fosterage systems (Chirwa 2002). From a child's point of
view, however, losing a parent is always a crisis, and taking in foster children
under duress can undoubtedly have adverse effects on them and their households, particularly when those households are impoverished. Whatever its
label, we have to recognize the ways that fostering has qualitatively changed
at a societal level under the impact of HIV/AIDS.

To understand how fostering is changing in modern times, kinship has to
reenter the debate at the organizational level, beyond the household, which is
often the analytic object of development studies (Notermans 2004; Madhavan 2004). While it is true that humanitarian intervention has also impacted
social traditions of fosterage, S. S. Hunter, recognizing the impending burden
of AIDS on traditional family fosterage in 1990, recommended continuing to
recognize the extended family as the most important source of support for
orphans and suggested aid programs to help build their capacity under crisis
(S. Hunter 1990). About twenty years later, the Joint Learning Initiative on
Children and HIV/AIDS (JLICA) reported, "Families and communities currently bear approximately 90% of the financial cost of caring for infected and
affected children in the areas hardest hit by aids. Many of these families are
already living in extreme poverty, yet few receive any support from sources
outside their communities" (Joint Learning Initiative on Children and HIV/
AIDS 2009, 2). This was the situation I encountered in my own fieldwork,
carried out at approximately the same time.

Orphans in our study were overwhelmingly cared for through kin networks, with only two of the thirty-nine children living with nonrelated care-givers. None relied primarily on institutions. Children were also still chang-ing households fairly frequently. Thirteen out of thirty-nine, or one-third, of the children moved to another household within the two years of the initial study (2007–9).

Grandmothers' Burden

As early as 1990, Janet and Philip Kilbride were claiming that, due to various socioeconomic factors, child care in East Africa was shifting toward grand-parents, who often end up taking care of children discarded by a daughter in favor of marrying a man who would not accept her children from a previ-ous marriage (Kilbride and Kilbride 1990, 189). Such was also the case for several children in the study group (see the appendix). In the age of HIV/AIDS, which has claimed not only parents but also aunts and uncles, grand-parents—and particularly grandmothers—are increasingly becoming the long-term caregivers for their grandchildren, and even their brothers' and sisters' grandchildren. In fact, most families' ranks have been so depleted by disease and economic hardship that there are few other options than to place orphaned children with grandparents. One grandmother in our study, Jaaja Rose, had taken in fourteen children after four of her eight children had passed away and three of the remaining four were bedridden with AIDS symptoms. Jaaja Rose knew some of the children might have gone to homes that were better off economically, but she has gladly taken them in, stating, "I'm afraid they would be mistreated by other relatives." With minimal eco-nomic support from family, friends, and neighbors, she felt she could watch over them and provide them with a loving environment.

Despite their sometimes fragile health and their limited ability to pro-vide monetarily for their children's children, many grandparents are doing the best they can at assuming the role of parents; and indeed, Tsilio Tamasane and Judith Head (2010) claim that children in grandparents' care suffer fewer disadvantages than initially believed by such organizations as the United Na-tions Children's Fund (UNICEF 2003). Still, grandparents face particular challenges in caring for a second generation. The sheer numbers of children being taken into grandparents' homes can put undue strain on already lim-ited household resources. The fact that older relatives are more likely to own arable land is an important consideration in placing orphans with them, yet the increase in household size can threaten that food security. In the peri-urban area where we conducted our study from 2007 to 2009, food security was rapidly being depleted: the area was essentially rural two decades earlier, and though elderly landholders still had plenty of land, they came under pressure to sell off parcels of it to people coming from the city looking for a quiet place to build a house. These people offered good money, so landholders sold off bits and pieces of their land for a handsome onetime fee. At the same time as landholders' property shrank, however, the number of dependents in their care increased, thus leaving them with too little land to adequately feed the growing household. The money would quickly run out, too, often leaving them more impoverished than before. Alternately, people like Jaaja Rose got permission from the landowners to farm on adjacent vacant lots, but before long, the same urban pressures made it too valuable to hold onto, so the owners sold it. The community now has more walled compounds than open fields—and more income disparity due to the influx of well-to-do new residents who bought land from impoverished longtime landowners.

Little of the literature on orphan care focuses much on the predicament of grandparents caring for AIDS-affected children. What few studies do consider them indicate that stress levels are particularly high among elderly caregivers (Oburu 2004). Preferring to detail biomedical ailments over emotional ones, many elderly caregivers we spoke with often cited their own "pressure" (i.e., high blood pressure) as a manifestation of their stressful situations. But this stoicism belies that fact that they too are suffering emotionally from the loss and dispersal of family, as well as the erosion of their own support base, due to HIV/AIDS (Swift and Maher 2008, 43). Having endured not only multiple bereavements and burdens due to AIDS and other shocks, many grandmothers are so busy trying to ensure their household members' survival that they themselves do not get time to mourn their own losses. Ailments such as "pressure" could thus be physical manifestations of such rapid and successive shifts between bereavement and providing care and support to others. Jaaja Rose, for example, had not only cared for more than a dozen children due to the deaths of her own children, but she has been palliative caregiver for multiple adult relatives who have passed away in her home, one after the other. When we caught up with her in 2012, a female relative in her care had just passed away. In addition, her brother (and father to the twins described in chapter 6), who had been bedridden for four years, was in her constant care. By then, he had gone blind and was showing signs of deterioration with which she and her household had become quite familiar. "Any day now . . ." she said to us in July, and in August, he passed away. Jaaja Rose reported the twins' distress at losing their father, but when asked how *she* was doing, Jaaja Rose tended to keep quiet and display little emotion, though as my assistant Faridah noted after leaving Jaaja Rose's house that day, "It's clear she is shaken by all the death around her."

Such "care fatigue" is becoming common among grandmothers, and it is compounded by the lack of attention (in what medical care exists) to psychological well-being (Parsons 2012, 106)—for children or their caregivers. This pattern may well have deleterious social effects beyond the household, as grandmothers too stressed at providing for so many with so little also have limited emotional resources to share. As Swift and Maher warn, "A nation that cannot grieve cannot move on, cannot affirm life and move into the future with a sense of optimism" (2008, 47). Jaaja Hamidah, grandmother to Justine and John (see chapter 6), told us, "First of all, people should know that raising an orphan isn't an easy thing, especially for us grandmothers. We are old, and the whole pain we have after losing our children still lives in our hearts, so at times looking at children of your children becomes unbearable. Secondly, people should learn to help not only their families or relatives but community as a whole."

Further, this changing care dynamic reveals rifts in intergenerational relationships that can be difficult to close, especially under such difficult circumstances: grandparents often report some trouble exacting the kinds of respect and obedience they have come to expect from children, especially as the children grow older, more rebellious, and at times more knowledgeable through schooling than their grandparents (Swift and Maher 2008, 48), which, in turn, compounds the grandparents' stress of caregiving. In one case in our study, an elderly woman was taking care of a *great*-grandchild whom her rebellious granddaughter in her care had dumped on her after getting pregnant at fourteen—or rather, he was often taking care of her, as she was frequently bedridden. While six-year-old Joel (see appendix) had a roof over his head and some food in the garden, he was primarily responsible for the household chores and cultivation, as well as school and his great-grandmother's care.

These responsibilities cause a sense of disillusionment among elderly caregivers, who said they had envisioned being provided *for* by their families at their age. They had looked forward to an old age surrounded by family, but one of rest and reverence by younger kin. Instead they were still acting as caregivers and providers, raising a second generation of children. However, recent studies indicate that care is gradually shifting in Uganda from grandparents to other relatives (Roby 2011, 15).

The fathers of the children in our study were either nominally or completely uninvolved in their children's upbringing, partly due to the trends that Kilbride and Kilbride (1990) identified, but AIDS deaths have also compounded this problem. Despite customary paternal kin obligations to care for children of their clans, we noticed a marked absence of men in children's lives. Next, I explore the reasons for and consequences of this trend.

The Waning of Paternal Kin Obligation—Just When It is Needed Most

In her criticism of anthropological studies of kinship, Janet Carsten (2004) argues for a focus on people, homes, and everyday practice rather than on groups, systems, and structures. Traditionally, "kinship obligations determine whether a child goes to maternal aunts, paternal aunts, grandmothers, or more distantly related kin. The choice of the foster parent also depends on the reasons for fostering" (Madhavan 2004, 1445). With the increase in "crisis fostering," however, there is as much motivation for kin to *avoid* fostering responsibilities as there is reason to claim orphans under rights and obligations to foster; poverty and the proliferation of orphans in the context of HIV/AIDS has overburdened many traditionally obliged to care for kin's children. Often missing from these studies are the viewpoints of the children who change homes as they lose their parents. Notermans cautions, "Anthropological studies [of fosterage], based on cultural ideals of African kinship, generally do not differentiate between the various members of the extended kinship network. By contrast, children do, and challenge the notion that parents care equally for all children in the kin network" (2008, 356–57). Here, I want to explore the significance of patriliny for orphans in Uganda, who are increasingly being raised by matrilineal kin (Roby 2011, 16).

While it is traditionally the obligation of the patrilineage to care for children who have lost their parents, it is also the patrilineal kin's prerogative to strategically claim or reject responsibility for children of their lineage. The ways children experience orphanhood and fostering therefore rest heavily on their biological mothers' life courses (Notermans 2008, 373), and more and more children are being fostered within maternal kin networks. In the context of HIV/AIDS and deepening poverty, moreover, patrilineal kin do not readily assume responsibility for the care of dependent children of their male kin until the mother has also died. If they do take in children at that point, it is not the men of the clan but the women who take on the work of orphan care. This caregiving role is imposed upon them by the husband's clan—usually without them being consulted. Such a situation may be where "evil stepmother" tropes gain salience in children's experiences (Cheney 2007b, 235–36): adults and children alike often said that women resent taking care of nonbiological children, but this resentment usually pertained more narrowly to children of their husband's previous or other wives. Oleke and colleagues have pointed out that "the 'wantedness' of orphans by their foster families is important in determining their well-being" (Oleke et al. 2006, 280). Castle's 1996 study of fostering in Mali found that children who were generally voluntarily fostered did not suffer any nutritional disadvantages, but those who were fostered out of necessity tended to become undernourished (as reported in Madhavan 2004). Orphans in Oleke's 2006 study in Uganda suffered disproportionately poorer care and higher labor exploitation in homes where "the inherently strained relationship between co-wives was often transferred to a deceased co-wife's children, i.e. to the orphans" (Oleke et al. 2006, 271–72). It may be for this reason that orphans in the care of paternal kin are not necessarily better off than those in the care of maternal kin. However, children who live with their mothers in a stepfather's household experience similar strains.

Pearl, an eight-year-old child in our study (see appendix), and her older sister, Sandra, lived with their mother and stepfather after their father had died and their mother had remarried. The stepfather made it clear that he did not want to take care of children who were not his; he did not even acknowledge their presence in his home, he took any opportunity he could to punish them, and he never helped with their school fees. The mother also neglected Pearl and Sandra to appease her husband, forcing them to sleep on mats in the storeroom. Their mother had since had more children with this husband, but he never let Pearl and Sandra even touch the things he brought home for his own children. Pearl therefore referred to them as "mother's kids" rather than her siblings, signaling her alienation. In her picture of her home, she excluded her stepfather and half siblings but included her father, in the form of a coffin. Though she drew several items that existed in the household, such as a bicycle (which her stepfather, a fishmonger, used as transport) and a cupboard, she also listed a number of things she wanted, such as a car or a television (fig. 10). On the other hand, a number of women whose male partners had died left their children with maternal or paternal female relatives so that they could move on to new relationships with other men—on which they were often financially dependent. Because, as Pearl's story demonstrates, the children of other men were not typically welcomed by stepfathers, these children were left behind, and in a few instances, their mothers ended communication with their children altogether (see children's profiles, e.g. Willy's, in the appendix for examples).

Even as they sometimes try to work around bloodline patriarchy—often to secure access to men's resources through their children—women's strategies can actually uphold that same patriarchy. Notermans's research on fosterage in Cameroon examines how the foster transaction enables women to construct and to strengthen matrilineal bonds; it yields them power and autonomy in society where patriliny operates simultaneously, and at certain moments in their lives even undermines their own freedom and power of decision (Notermans 2004, 51). One way women in Uganda try to work around patriarchal constraints is to maintain care for their maternal kin's children—

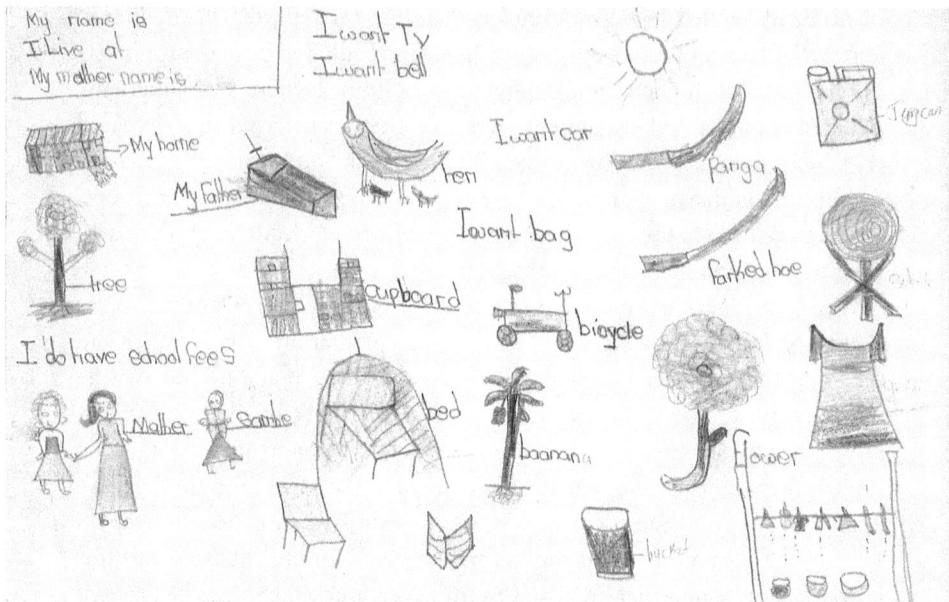

FIGURE 10. Pearl's drawing of her home. Her stepfather and half siblings are excluded while she, her mother, and her sister remain in the lower left corner. Her deceased father is also included in the upper left, in the form of a coffin.

from whom they can derive some household assistance and/or who they hope will one day reciprocate—while also trying to remind patrilineal kin of their obligations in order to receive assistance from the patrilineal clans of children in their care. Maternal grandmothers, for example, might try to claim their daughters' children by acknowledging paternity but refusing to accept bride wealth from the children's father or preventing them from sign-ing a child's birth certificate—in other words, evoking the rules of patriarchy to resist it. This situation also sometimes happens by default, as a decline in formal marriage and increase in children born out of wedlock has accompa-nied—and even predated (Kilbride and Kilbride 1990)—the onslaught of the AIDS pandemic. Oleke, Blystad, and Rekdal's study found that 63 percent of orphans surveyed in northern Uganda "were found to be no longer headed by resourceful paternal kin in a manner deemed culturally appropriate by the patrilineal Langi society, but rather by marginalised widows, grandmothers or other single women receiving little support from the paternal clan" (2005, 2628). While the numbers in our study were not quite that high, the trend toward matrilocal care was likewise apparent, with just over half the children in the study living with maternal relatives. Further, fathers and other pater-nal kin tend to put up next to no resistance to claims by maternal relatives, which effectively releases paternal kin from any obligation to provide materially for the child. In fact, paternal and maternal relatives increasingly claim that young children especially are better off with the maternal clan, albeit for ostensibly different developmental reasons. Indeed, many orphans themselves claim that they feel well cared for by maternal relatives (Oleke et al. 2006, 273). The effect of this consensus, however, is that maternal relatives have more and more trouble making successful claims for material support from the patrilineal clans, leaving maternal aunts, grandparents, and other predominantly female kin in relative poverty as their influence on community resource allocation also weakens (Oleke, Blystad, and Rekdal 2005). This is one factor that may contribute to the "feminization of poverty" in rural Africa (Kabadaki 2001), with female-headed households having become one of the biggest indicators of child poverty (Fussell and Greene 2002, 47). Such patterns reinforce the need to empower both women and children, but patriarchal privilege continues to bind them. There was a consensus among caregivers in our study that orphans suffer more today than when they were growing up because it is harder both to provide for them and to integrate them into paternal extended family. Despite some room to maneuver, these cultural systems work against women whose caregiving strategies can play into the hands of patriarchal power; they cannot win in a system when they have no rights to make claims on fathers to help support children, but they can also have those children taken away from them because even when a woman raises a child alone, the children still "belong" to the father's clan and even as social ties with paternal kin wane, the concept of shared blood continues to dominate notions of kinship affiliation.

Orphans' Identities and Mobility across Family Ties

Children, as persons moving between homes, offer us a way of grasping the significance of kinship from the inside by exploring the everyday intimacies that occur there.
JANET CARSTEN (2004, 56)

Blood as an idiom of relatedness gains poignant significance only in orphans' and others' imaginings of their kin identities, perhaps because blood ties are so palpably threatened by AIDS and orphanhood. It is therefore important to ask what effects this transformation of kinship will have on orphaned children and their family networks as they grow. Aside from material deprivation through the maternalization of care and the feminization of poverty (fig. 11), orphans living with maternal kin can quickly lose touch with the paternal clans with whom they hope to identify. Though people on all sides tend to

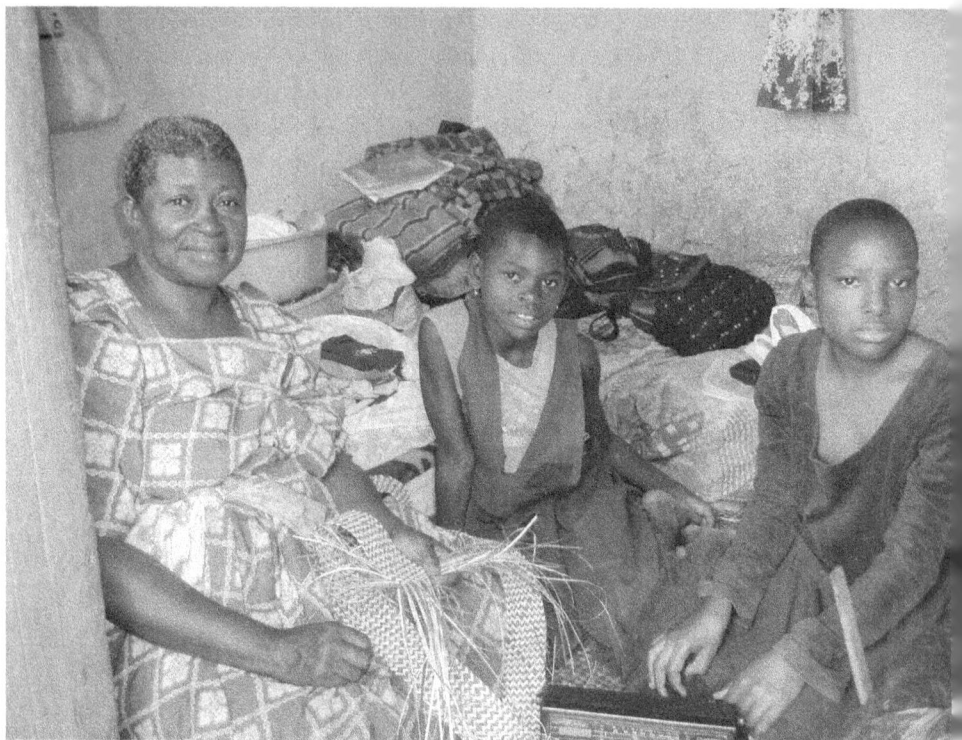

FIGURE 11. A grandmother and the two grandchildren she cares for live together in a one-room apartment.

think young children will do better when being cared for on the mother's side, a number of older children in our study expressed a desire to return to their father's kin so they would "know their family." Orphans thus shifted over time from matrilineal kin's homes in early childhood to patrilineal kin's homes once they reached adolescence and young adulthood and chose to go live with them—and as patrilineal kin who had previously been absent in their lives returned to make claims on their kin. The idea of "blood" as a bonding substance legitimizes claims of "ownership" by virtue of kinship— but typically only when the father's family chooses to activate it. Women and matrilineal clan members do not have the same prerogative.

At the same time that many paternal clans ask to have their adolescent "sons and daughters" back, orphans' ideas of "home" become imbued with symbolic value as these young people formulate their identities. Despite being initially rejected by patrilineal family and raised by matrilineal family members, orphans may want to go live with their patrilineal family as they grow older due to the notion of shared "blood" and the importance of clan association to young people's identity formation. The gender of the children themselves influences how they relate to kin. One family's story ably illustrates these trends—and what sometimes happens as a result.

Olivia cared for her sister until the sister's death in 2004 (see appendix). Before passing away, her sister had asked Olivia to care for her three children after she died, since parents and direct siblings—and especially sisters born of the same mother—are considered the most reliable foster parents for orphans. The fact that Olivia had cared for her sister, and by extension her children, throughout her illness also eased the children's transition after their mother's death. Because their aunt already lived with them, she simply assumed full responsibility after her sister became too ill. Such close nurturing ties explain why children mostly have no difficulty adapting to foster families with whom they are used to frequent contact from birth (Notermans 2008, 361). It was also a smoother transition for them because the siblings were not split up or forced to move from the home they had shared with their mother and aunt into new households.

At the time, Olivia was studying at the university to be a teacher, with the help of a German sponsor. None of the paternal clans of the children's three fathers stepped forward to offer to care for the children when their mother died, though Olivia continued to solicit support from them anyway. When that failed, she also went to her own relatives. A maternal uncle responded by paying their school fees for a while, but he went to Sudan on business in 2008 and they lost contact with him. The fees were not paid, and the children had all dropped out of school by the end of 2008. Around this time, both Olivia's eleven-year-old niece Agatha and fourteen-year-old nephew Jacob started expressing desires to connect with their "real" (fathers') clans.[2]

When their uncle disappeared and stopped paying fees, Olivia—who had finished her teaching certificate but still had not found a job—appealed again to the children's paternal kin to help support the children's education. In Agatha's instance, the father's family said they would not help unless the girl came to live with them, but Olivia hesitated to relinquish her; she did not wish to break her promise to her sister, but, as Fiona Bowie points out, "In many African societies, as elsewhere in the world, to refuse to give a child to someone who has a culturally validated right to ask for it is considered selfish and normally blameworthy" (2004, 11). Besides, Olivia was struggling to finish a teaching degree and get a job that would help her to manage care for both her own young son (whose father was also entirely absent) and the two nephews and a niece she was trying to support. So if she was fatigued physically, emotionally, and financially by caring for the children, she was also being given a convenient excuse to pass child care on to the traditionally obliged paternal kin. Agatha herself was also motivated both by the opportunity to continue with school and to get acquainted with her paternal clan.

When Agatha visited her father's family over the 2008–9 holiday (November to January), they asked her directly to come live with them. Girls of Agatha's age are often treasured by the patrilineal clan for the bride-price they can bring in once they marry, and their chastity is well protected to fetch an even higher bride-price.[3] Olivia suspected that this was partly their motivation, but they told her that if Agatha lived with them, she would go to school again, and she accepted, so Olivia let her go. They kept their promise to put her in school.

Boys have different concerns with paternal clans that have more to do with questions of identity. The issue of clan identification was especially important for boys coming of age, not merely for purposes of establishing their identities but for the ways that recognition by the clan would later enable them to inherit family resources that move through the male line. Jacob, Olivia's fourteen-year-old nephew, also dropped out of school in 2008 when his uncle stopped paying his fees. Though he had known of his father's family in Masaka, he had never met them, and his peers even teased him about it. For this reason, he too spent his 2008–9 holidays with his father's family to get acquainted with them. Olivia said he came back changed, talking a lot about family and the importance of kin identity. He said he realized that his patrilineal clan and father's family were important in his life. Though none of them had stepped up to care for him when his father died, they told him now that he *really* belonged with them. When he knew that he would not be going to school anyway, he asked to go live with them, stressing that it was essential to him as a boy "to know who he was." Olivia gave her permission.

Nyambedha and Aagaard-Hansen have noted, "When children find themselves placed under the direct control of adult members of the extended family, they return to the social position of being children responding purely to the demands of childhood. Children's places in such situations are seen as processes that are firmly grounded in social interactions, available support networks and opportunities within the community" (2003, 173). In choosing to return to their fathers' families, then, Agatha and Jacob were not only assuming their proper places as dependent (and subservient) children within their patrilineages but also hoping to gain the entitlements that come with such belonging. The establishment of a clan identity was particularly important to Jacob in constructing his ethnic and gendered identity as a Muganda male. If a Muganda father does not know where he came from and has a child, then he effectively cannot give the child a name because he can only guess his own clan affiliation. When women have children out of wedlock, by contrast, they usually choose a surname from the alleged father's clan, whether he accepts the child as his or not. It may be the only way that women can eventually make a claim of support, however weak, from the father's family.

In another instance wherein a boy was raised solely by his mother after the father refused to acknowledge paternity, the mother was always telling her son who his father was. So once the boy grew up and started to succeed at business, he used that success to try to claim his own way back into the father's clan. He would show up uninvited to family activities and try to keep in touch, bringing gifts to remind them that he was ready to be there when they needed him. This was his way of trying to claim his identity as a man, despite his father's clan's perpetual rejection of his claim that he belonged to them.

Boys are also motivated to secure the entitlements attendant with belonging to the paternal clan, most especially inheritance of land. Our study found, however, that as young male orphans grew to adulthood in maternal homes, they experienced problems inheriting property from their deceased fathers' clans, though they are customarily entitled to it—and this conflict often caused young men a great deal of stress. Elizabeth Cooper (2010) has explored how traditional inheritance patterns have important yet little-understood implications for the intergenerational transmission of poverty in sub-Saharan Africa—in terms of both inclusion and exclusion—particularly for orphans. Hence the need for orphans to establish relations with paternal kin as early as possible to ensure fulfillment of their culturally expected social support.

As with Agatha's paternal relatives, Olivia doubted Jacob's paternal clan's intentions; she suspected that, now that Jacob was older, maybe they were only claiming him because they could get him to work.[4] Many maternal caregivers like Olivia noted that although paternal kin often refused care of young children of their clans, they typically reversed that decision and asked for children when they reached late childhood or early adolescence. They suspected the patrilineal clan of claiming entitlements to the children's labor once they were old enough to contribute to a rural household's workload. With 41 percent of African children under age fourteen working, particularly in domestic tasks, Oleke and colleagues have noted that "the local communities justify the involvement of children in domestic labour as normal preparation for the future, and do not mention the abuse and exploitation that is nearly always inherent. This is more dominant in the case of orphans, who are often removed from school to work in the field or home or to pursue outside employment to earn money for the family's survival" (Oleke et al. 2006, 281). However, Jacob had determined before going to live with his father's family that he wanted to go to vocational school to learn to be a mechanic, so his Aunt Olivia helped him with the initial fees. While his father's family tolerated this continued education, they were not pleased because they had indeed expected him to contribute to the agricultural workload. They were glad that he helped on weekends and holidays, but they never gave him any of the income that was earned from the sale of the family farm's produce, and they refused to contribute any of that money to his vocational training.

Because of his desire to associate with his paternal kin, then, Jacob found himself inadvertently reinforcing the patrilineal ideal that allows for labor exploitation of children like him. For two and a half years, he worked on the family's farm, and his relatives kept the money he earned without so much as buying him clothes or adequately feeding him. He would pick up odd jobs at area garages to earn enough to buy his own clothes. His paternal grandfather welcomed him and would tell him stories about funny things his father did when he was alive or point out how Jacob was like his father, who had died when Jacob was five years old. Jacob also got along with his eldest cousin, but "the others didn't treat me like I was part of them," Jacob said, "almost like a lesser class, in fact." He was not sure exactly why they were threatened—the only thing he ever asked for was the use of his father's old bicycle to get to his vocational classes—but he felt constant discrimination there, down to the lesser amount and quality of food he was typically given at meals.

Jacob finally left in 2012 after being paid directly at a garage where he had been working for several weeks. He was not finding permanent work, and anyway, the tensions with his father's family were getting to be too much. Jacob took the money and returned to his Aunt Olivia's home in rags. He started looking for work in town, but Kampala garages tended not to value his certificate from a Masaka vocational school, and in any case they preferred to hire someone with experience. He would have to pay four hundred thousand Ugandan shillings (about 240 US dollars) just for the opportunity to apprentice at a garage, and he did not have such resources. Instead, he went to Juba, Sudan, to join his maternal uncle, who was operating a *matatu* (minibus shuttle) there. Jacob was the *matatu's* conductor for eight months, and though he had hoped to make enough money in Juba to raise the money for a mechanics apprenticeship, Juba was so expensive that anything he made went into his own upkeep. When the *matatu* broke down, Jacob returned to Kampala empty-handed. When we caught up with Jacob in 2014 at twenty years old, he was living with his maternal grandmother near to his Aunt Olivia's house and was earning occasional income as a day laborer at construction sites, usually carrying bricks for the builders. For this he sometimes got ten thousand Ugandan shillings (about six US dollars) per day, but the work was too inconsistent to save money. His dream, though, was still to be a mechanic.

Agatha, by contrast, had completed her Senior Six (college prep) exams by 2014 at age seventeen and had qualified for university admission. Her paternal aunt and uncle had treated her throughout as their own child, and they were trying to raise the money to send her on to the university. Jacob surmised it was because her father had left only daughters and no sons, so she was not seen as a threat to the family's resources; in fact, she might indeed bring them wealth. "They always think that boys will come to claim support, though girls can leave anytime, and the family gets bride wealth," Jacob pointed out. "Boys, on the other hand, require assistance to raise bride wealth." Agatha also lived closer to her Aunt Olivia and her maternal grandmother than Jacob had while he was in Masaka, so she never took more than a month without coming to visit them.

Such incidents raise the concern that in the midst of dwindling resources, relatives sometimes make (gendered) decisions about who will care for orphans based more on their own self-interest than on the best interests of the children. Often, negotiations over who will care for children in the wake of their caregiver's death circulate around not only questions of which households have the capacity to take in more orphans, but which child will be of the most use—or the least trouble—to the adult head of household. "I'll take Prossy because she's quiet and a hard worker," an aunt or uncle may say, "But I don't want her brother; he's disobedient." This is another means through which many children end up with elderly grandparents. It is also a means through which siblings often get split up.

A relative's willingness to host an orphan is a conditional agreement; orphans must ingratiate themselves to caregivers, usually through daily exercise of obedience (*mpisa*).[5] When asked about the texture of their daily lives, most orphans rattled off an extensive list of the chores they were expected to do both before and after school—including farming, laundry, cooking, washing dishes, and caring for younger children in the household. At times, completing chores meant being late to school or missing it altogether. Children who do not conform to such adult expectations risk being cast out, especially after the benefits of enrollment in an orphan care program have been received or have ended. Obedience thus becomes a condition for care, reinforcing the usefulness of children for their guardians.

This family dynamic leaves children exposed to greater and greater exploitation within their caregivers' homes—whether they are relatives or not. In one extreme case, two children in the study had been taken from a rural area to the home of a woman in the study community who claimed to be their grandmother but who was not actually related at all. She wanted some assistance with chores in her home and had assured the family in her home village that she could secure free schooling for the orphans from the community school near the city. When they refused to do chores, however, she kept them home from school. Their high rate of absenteeism alerted the head teacher, who investigated. She found that the woman had finally returned them to their home after they kept running away and sleeping at a neighbor's house.

"Blood Always Finds Its Way Home": The Significance of Patrilineal Identification for Orphans

To understand dynamics of child circulation requires a better grasp of the idiom of "blood," both as a metaphor of relatedness and as a substance that actually binds kin. In Buganda, as in many other sub-Saharan African belief systems, blood ties override any other kind of conceptualization of kinship. Both the mother and father contribute blood to the children, but the father's is considered somewhat stronger. Yet women, mothers and *ssengas* (advisorial paternal aunts), are the only ones who can curse a Baganda child—a sort of check on patriarchal power. In the Luganda language, people commonly talk about "blood" as an interchangeable word for the concept of kinship and kin themselves. For example, a granny may talk about wanting to care for a child "because s/he's my daughter's blood." In the age of HIV/AIDS, grandmothers may actually choose to take in orphaned children because these grandchildren can come to represent, through their "blood," their own missing children. Sometimes the grandchildren are all that the grandparent may have left of his or her deceased child. One grandmother who told me she took in her four granddaughters because they represent the blood of her dead daughter had even refused requests to give the children to their father's clan because, she said, "I couldn't watch my blood suffer" if they went to live with the father's family (fig. 12; see also Schatz 2007).

Blood is mainly operationalized in kinship systems through the ways it supposedly acts as a magnet to draw "its own" back to the clan. Powerful beliefs about blood demonstrate its significance as a tie that binds children to their patrilineage—even when paternity is not clearly established. When I asked my youth research assistants about it in a data analysis workshop, the proverb "Blood finds its way home" came up, meaning that children estranged from their fathers' clans are instinctually pulled back into the clans through their shared substance/kinship. Youth RA Sumayiya gave an example: if two men are fighting over the paternity of a woman's child, people often believe that the child will find its way back to its biological father, regardless of whom the mother may claim is the father. The father or his family can even use witchcraft to put a spell on the child, who will sicken until he or she is either reunited with the father or dies. I asked what happened if the father did not

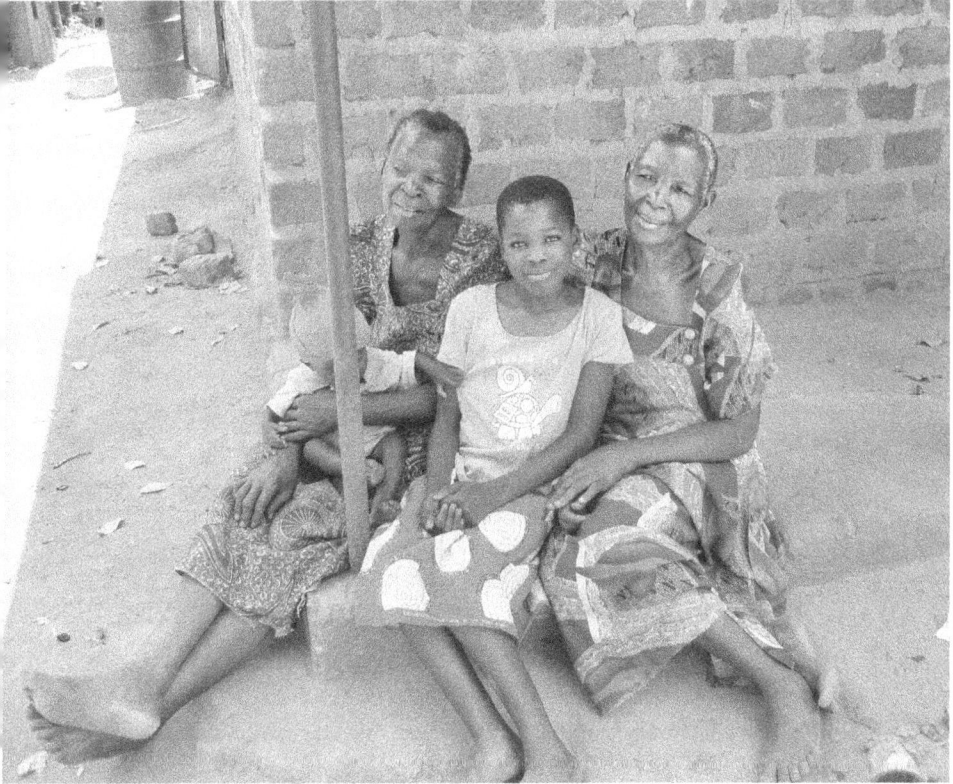

FIGURE 12. A maternal grandmother (*right*) sits with her twin sister and her granddaughter, one of the four granddaughters and a great-grandchild in her care. She prefers that her grandchildren stay with her because through their blood, they connect her to the daughter she has lost.

claim the child, and Sumayiya said that people believed that children would still find their way back to their paternal clan. She even said that people talk about blood as having a "smell" and that children know instinctually to whom they are related. Faridah thought Sumayiya translated the notion of "smelling" blood a little bit too literally. *Kusika* can mean "to pull" or "to inhale," among other things. But Faridah seconded the notion that children who are separated from their father will fall sick until they are reunited, sometimes due to witchcraft, or, as Sumayiya put it, "those local, local beliefs."

While witchcraft and kinship are closely linked in many cultures across Africa (Geschiere 2003), witchcraft often emerges in children's stories as a central concern in kin relations as well as a means of expressing the domestic tensions and conflicts in which they sometimes find themselves embroiled (Notermans 2008, 358). Faridah knew a child who was taken to the United Kingdom by her mother and fell sick until she returned to her father's clan's

land in Uganda. Faridah also raised the example of twins, who are highly re-
vered in Baganda culture and who therefore must be brought to their father's
courtyard. Sometimes the traditions differ by family, but many people seem
to believe that staying with the father's side is actually a matter of life and
death.

There was some disagreement among the youth RAs about how strong
this notion of blood is among the Baganda and other Ugandan ethnic groups.
Youth RA Michael (who is Langi) thought it depended on whether you were
brought up "in civilization or tradition." Since Michael and Jill grew up with
weak ties to extended family and do not have strong ties to their natal villages,
they did not feel held by those beliefs. Michael personally did not feel drawn
by any ritual, or even the death of a relative. He agreed that such beliefs were
the realm of the peasant, though some people who live in Kampala will even
say that you have to take a child back to their village to be blessed by the grannies, or it can negatively affect children as they grow up and their attachments
to distant relatives are not reinforced. Jill said that she had seen that happen
to people who were dedicated to a relative as an infant.

James, a Pokot on his father's side and a Muganda on his mother's, chimed
in that "blood" was an important notion that certainly played into his experience after his father died in 2001 (Cheney 2007b, 98). Both his Baganda and
Pokot relatives related any suffering James and his family experienced to the
broken blood link his father's death represented. They thought his suffering
would lessen as he went back to his father's village and got to know his paternal side of the family. His paternal relatives, whom he had never known—
since he grew up in Kampala and not his father's rural homestead—promised
to look after him and his siblings, taught them tribal rituals, and gave them
some articles of his father's, including his old clothes. But they suspected that
James and his siblings may have been having trouble because they had not
gone through the usual rites of passage. Like Jacob, James's older brother has
gone back on his own and spent some time, and he recommends that all of
them go and get to know that side of the family. "But I don't think that this is
so necessary for the suffering of someone," James concluded. "What I believe
is that when someone produces a child and runs away with the child and the
man is unaware . . . I think that's when those things have to come in."

All of these stories reflect the extent to which blood, despite its potential
to act destructively as a carrier of pathogens, is also seen as a substance that
immutably binds people in kin relations. In fact, I surmise that strengthened
belief in blood as an affective "adhesive" of kin bonds may be of such importance to AIDS-affected children and caregivers precisely *because* it counter-
acts the discourses of blood as the carrier of the HIV/AIDS virus—which also

runs through families (and particularly through mother-to-child transmission) and threatens to break them asunder. Seen in the context of the AIDS pandemic and socioeconomic constraints, provision of child care increasingly hinges on the attendant obligations of these blood ties. For orphans who may find it more of a challenge under current circumstances, then, their stakes in establishing blood ties, particularly with patrilineal kin, may be even greater. In terms of everyday care—even when met with skepticism—people hedge their bets by invoking blood ties to ensure a child's well-being. Orphans and their maternal caregivers alike thus try to secure paternal care by demanding adherence to blood's cultural scripts.

Shifting Notions of "Home"

While very young and/or newly orphaned children might have little say in their household placement, I have shown that this situation changes as they grow. Orphans' choices to go live with paternal kin at a certain age reflect their active engagement in constructing their own notions of "home" through the powerful metaphor of blood and, more broadly by extension, their proper place in the world where they are otherwise at more risk of being considered "rootless" because of their orphanhood. To establish their place in the paternal kin network however, they have to navigate some of the difficult cultural politics mentioned earlier in this chapter, much of which points to the distinction Pierre Bourdieu (1977) made between "official" and "practical" kinship. Much of the literature on kinship and home centers on the hearth, with food as the primary substance that binds children to caregivers through feeding and sharing of other resources (Carsten 2004, 35). John Borneman (2001) similarly centers discussion around care. This focus would make orphans "practically" members of the maternal clans that take care of them—but while this view may be true to some extent, it presents a static vision of the nature of kinship ties that can and do change over time. It also empties children of their agency to choose—even if that choice is to fulfill a preexisting cultural script. Notermans points out that "as kinship evolves in homes through sharing food and intimacy, children directly experience how kinship is created, disputed and defined and how lived kinship is inextricably linked with mobility, flexibility and power dynamics" (Notermans 2008, 355). In addition, the idea of "home" invokes emotional affiliations based on active, imaginative refigurings of belonging that might mitigate their marginalization, particularly as orphaned children. However much children may feel a sense of belonging in the homes of their maternal kin, then, their desire to identify with their patrilineal clan may lead them to migrate to their father's family. Jacob felt this pull enough to go and spend two and a half years of his adolescence with a family that ended up not caring for him well. Jacob even took his younger brother Hakim to visit his father's family in 2013 (both their fathers' families live in Masaka) so he could get to know his "blood" relatives. They also wanted Hakim to stay—"We want our son," they kept saying—but after Jacob's experience, Aunt Olivia refused to let Hakim go, out of concern that he too would automatically drop out of school and start working their land if he went there. "At that age, they like them because they can still get them to do anything," Jacob and Olivia said. And though Jacob was satisfied that he learned enough about himself while staying with his father's family, he can never dream of going back there now. People will say, "Now you know where you will be buried!" but he does not even want to be buried there or want to inherit any part of the estate. Thus, multiple factors weigh into children's and caregivers' decisions, and that "by initiating, ending and reinitiating fosterage, children actively construct their life between different competing kin groups" (Notermans 2008, 367).

Youth RA Sumayiya's movement between households as a child demonstrates this pattern as well: her parents divorced when she was two years old, and she lived with her father until his death when she was six years old. Her mother took her into her home then, but as she had no regular work, Sumayiya dropped out of school. She spent several years moving around with her mother, and suffering abuses from her mother's boyfriends, by whom her mother had more children. When she heard at age twelve that her paternal uncle (who was already caring for several other extended family members) was willing to pay for her school fees, she left her mother's home and went to live with her aunt and uncle. Sumayiya's choice to pursue education through her father's kin, but also her uncle's patrilineal kin obligation, facilitated her return to her father's family (and to school) after six years.

"Fictive" Kinship Revisited

The intermittent nature of care can leave children with little option but to try to cultivate kin relationships with unrelated but well-meaning adults, including anthropologists, from whom they might supplement the limited support they get from their de facto caregivers. According to Jeffrey Kaufmann and Annie Phillippe Rabodoarimiadana, "Being cast as 'one of theirs,' as a fictive family member, is a way in which informants . . . become imbedded in historical and anthropological fieldwork. . . . This practice of making kin out of thin air, so to speak, is less a projection of the fieldworker, who has in many cases come to the field from afar, and more an extension of practices by informants or hosts" (2003, 182). Where children find blood ties lacking in social practice, they may also actively create them: for example, youth RA Malik called me "Mum" as a means to secure support in the absence of his biological mother. Strategies of "fictive" or "social" kinship thus also need to be revisited, as orphaned children may deploy it to gain the entitlements of particular kin relationships. In fact, even the terminology of "fictive" kinship has come into question, as anthropologists studying kinship have questioned the strictly biological models of kinship in favor of defining relatedness as "the process of caring and being cared for" (Borneman 2001, 31; Carsten 2004). For this reason, I prefer to use the term *social kinship*.

Malik had taken to calling me "Mum" after I started providing his school fees, confiding at one point, "I lost my mother when I was very young, but you do all those things that a mother would do for me." I was flattered by the honorific, but I was soon to learn that I was not the only one he called "Mum": when Malik's dance troupe was to perform at his brother's wedding reception in 2007, I arrived early with him while they were still setting up. He led me over to where two of his aunts were tying ribbons and attaching them to the floral arrangements. He introduced me to them, and while I sat with them making bows, Malik continued to set up the band. Imagine his embarrassment when he rushed over shouting, "Mum! Mum!" and both his two aunts and I turned around! My jaw dropped in disbelief for a moment, but as I got over my own (mild) sense of betrayal (it is quite common to call aunties—and grandmothers—"Mum," as the word for each of these relatives is often the same in local vernacular languages), I realized that the cultivation of relationships with several different "mums" was actually a brilliant survival strategy on Malik's part; such deliberate assignment of kinship terms by orphans raises the possibility of transformative relationships: by calling someone "Mum," a child elicits "discourse expectations" of appropriate care and support from a variety of adults (Urban 1996, 131). From several aunties to other potential benefactors such as me, Malik had likely racked up quite a number of surrogate parents willing to support him in various ways. The success of this strategy hinged on the recognition of both affective and material elements that are essential to local constructions of kinship, and which international development's approaches to the AIDS orphan crisis tend to gloss over, or even subvert. This oversight gives anthropologists and development practitioners alike occasion to revisit social kinship as a conscious construction by orphans in contradiction to local norms—and as a cultural process that "addresses contemporary social issues, and reflects anthropology's current concerns with process, variation, and history" (Stone 2001, 10).

Orphans' Circulation Strategies in the Context of
Changing Paternal Foster Obligations

I have shown how notions of "blood"—and particularly patrilineage—continue to play an important symbolic role in orphaned children's imaginations of "home" and their sense of social belonging in Uganda. Yet, despite the continued importance of "blood" as an idiom of relatedness and "home" as a place tied to the patrilineage, the presence of paternal kin in orphaned children's lives is waning as more paternal clans relinquish their traditional obligations to absorb orphans, leaving the responsibility to maternal kin who may have less access to community resources. We have seen a few examples illustrating that orphans raised by maternal kin tend to revert to the "official" (or we might say ideal) kin narrative by identifying with their paternal clans, thus actively—if inadvertently—influencing the transformation of kinship. One of the practical consequences that we see already from this trend is that it leaves the maternal kin that provide for orphans earlier in life without later support in exchange for having raised those children—thus deepening maternal caregivers' poverty while also obviating the reciprocal relationships that have historically motivated fosterage. For all their efforts, though, some children in our study who changed households in search of greater stability and resources within their kin groups were still living hand to mouth, and their situations sometimes even worsened due to exploitation of their labor in the paternal kin's homes. Jacob's experience described in this chapter is one example of such an instance. The inconsistency between ideological constructions of kinship and the realities facing orphans can thus sometimes even work to the detriment of their own and other OVC's well-being by reinforcing the very patriarchal privilege that marginalizes maternal caregivers while letting paternal relatives off the hook for their familial duties.

While Carsten claims that anthropological studies of bodily substance "challenge any simple dichotomy between idioms of a bounded individual body/person and immutable kinship relations in Euro-American contexts and more fluid, mutable bodies and relations elsewhere" (2011, 19), I would caution against dismissing the enduring symbolic power of "blood ties" for orphaned children in the age of HIV/AIDS. The ambivalence that characterizes the situation of orphans has already instigated cultural changes that increase orphan's vulnerability. It is precisely because these kinship ties are being threatened by AIDS and its related social effects that Ugandans, from orphaned children to their caregivers, emphasize the idiom of blood as an immutable connection with kin in a world of uncertainty. The structural context of poverty also cannot be ignored in this context, as orphans' kin typically do not wish to be relieved of their filial duties so much as of their poverty. In this situation, Abebe and Aase are right to call for "research that draws on the perspectives of the children, and challenges the taken-for-granted premises that orphans are burdens not resources, is crucial" (2007, 2068). It is also important to maintain fluid, processual understandings of children's active constructions of kinship (Notermans 2008, 373), and throughout the life course. Bringing anthropological and development studies of fostering together with children's studies' concern for understanding children's perspectives helps draw attention to the dynamic aspects of kinship as well as the way children's concerns shape them. Understanding kinship as a process of imagining as well as material practice highlights the contradictory effects of AIDS orphanhood, in which the pull of patrilineal "blood" weakens reciprocity for maternal care—and even allows for exploitation of orphaned children. This approach may in turn lead to capacity-building interventions that better account for the intergenerationality of negotiated kin care networks, as well as orphaned children's own motivations for moving across family networks, thereby creating avenues for better material and affective support of children as they find their way "home" in an uncertain world.

8

Orphanhood and the Politics of Adoption in Uganda

As I sat at the Kampala babies' home I visited while doing fieldwork in 2009, I fell into conversation with Vitale Mukasa, the Ugandan parent of a child he and his wife had recently adopted there. He beamed with pride at the thought of his new daughter, a little girl named Carol.[1] Given his obvious pride in her, I was surprised when he then casually volunteered, "We don't want to tell anyone she's adopted, so we just tell people she's a child from an extramarital affair of mine."

"*That's* a better story!?" I gasped.

He nodded resolutely, looking me straight in the eye: "*That's* a better story."

I was not prepared for the stigma that surrounded domestic adoption in Uganda. The extent to which Mukasa, for example, found it easier to claim that his adopted child had been born out of wedlock than to admit that they had formally adopted her seemed out of step with the widespread practice of informal fostering of children that I had been studying for several years at that point. Despite a proliferation of orphans due to the AIDS pandemic, few African countries until recently have encouraged adoption, domestic or international, as a response. Though AIDS infection rates peaked in Uganda in the early 1990s, the government resisted intercountry adoption, which was becoming more popular at the time as a means of dealing with the consequent "orphan crisis" that threatened to overwhelm extended-family care. But the same fostering traditions and beliefs about "blood" as a substance that not only binds kin but also carries pathogens such as AIDS and certain moral character traits make formal adoption of unrelated children rare in Uganda. Nonetheless, there are strong sentiments against foreigners adopting Ugandan children, for fear the children may lose touch with their Ugandan heritage or, worse, experience abuse and maltreatment. This situation leaves abandoned and institutionalized orphans in a double "blood bind," where on the one hand, they are nobody's children, but on the other, they are *Uganda's* children.

The same powerful beliefs about "blood" and kinship that draw orphans to paternal clans thus also impact the growing adoption movement in Uganda. In this chapter, I return to the broader national and international context to consider how "blood" as a metaphor of relatedness has prevented domestic adoption from playing a greater role in responses to orphanhood. At the same time, intercountry adoption as a globalized mode of reproduction is fixing its focus on Uganda, thus challenging Ugandan *blood binds*—the moral and political economies—of orphan care. Recent debates have yielded a quagmire of tensions and contradictions surrounding Ugandan attitudes about adoption. My goal here is not necessarily to resolve these contradictions but rather to inhabit them to see what they reveal about kinship, politics, and belonging where child care and protection are concerned. To do so, I borrow Didier Fassin's notion of moral economy. Drawing from earlier conceptualizations by E. P. Thompson and James Scott, Fassin uses the term *moral economy* to describe the values and norms that inform common moral worlds and "the moral evaluation of difference" (Fassin 2005, 366). Because, as Fassin points out, "a bureaucracy can become 'emotional,'" moral economy helps get at the "moral heart" of policies (2005, 366) such as child care and protection. More recently Fassin has also suggested that "the problematization of childhood in contemporary societies . . . has to do . . . with the sort of moral truth through which we construct children—not only in our familiar environment but also in far-off lands" (2013, 111). Few international policy issues thus get more "emotional" than intercountry adoption as a means of building—and sometimes tearing apart—families. I therefore wish to consider here how kinship—biological and social—enters debates about the political economy of adoption as a mode of family production.

First, I summarize the moral and political economies of intercountry adoption that have led to its recent dramatic increase in Uganda; then I discuss the moral economy of child abandonment and increasing institutionalization in Uganda and explain why domestic adoption has been rare. Finally, I consider how the broader moral and political economies of intercountry adoption are confronting the moral economy of kinship and belonging within Uganda.

Intercountry Adoption in Global Context

Even before the establishment of the Victorian workhouses on which Charles Dickens based his novel *Oliver Twist*, orphanhood in Europe and the United States was predominantly defined as a social rather than a biological category. Though often represented as parentless and abandoned, poor European children were commonly placed temporarily in institutions by their impoverished parents or law enforcement as a stopgap measure, to be retrieved when their parents' circumstances improved. At the conjuncture of the rise of the modern welfare state and the changing conceptions of children as precious and priceless (Zelizer 1985), social orphans of the poor—because they were seen as innocent but also able to be reformed—were separated by institutionalization from their parents, who were thereby excluded from citizenship (Murdoch 2006). Though institutionalization of children of the poor has fallen out of favor in the Global North—and in development prescriptions for children due to its deleterious effects on children's well-being—the establishment of orphanages (often by Western charities) is ironically seen as an appropriate charitable response to orphanhood in the Global South, and parents are likewise using it as a stopgap coping mechanism for child care in lean economic times. Yet because the same type of reification of orphans has now gone global through international regimes of humanitarianism, people continue to assume that children in institutions are parentless (Bartholet and Smolin 2012), or that a parentless child also means that a child has no family or community. Now as then, such is rarely the case; but whereas children are seen as worthy of assistance, they are similarly targeted for help while their guardians are excluded.

While the shifting frontier of intercountry adoption ostensibly reflects a concern with child rescue (Davies 2011), intercountry adoption is usually spurred more by demand—amid falling fertility rates and availability of adopted children in the United States and Europe—than by supply of orphans needing homes (Cheney and Rotabi 2014). Despite this, the idea that orphans need "saving" through intercountry adoption has persisted since the Korean War of the 1950s (Marre and Briggs 2009, 8). Global media coverage has brought awareness of such crises to potential adopters (Cartwright 2005; Hoffman 2012), and the Internet has facilitated the networking of potential transnational adoptive parents with agencies, orphanages, and other facilitators around the world (Marre and Briggs 2009, 13). Demand for intercountry adoption is thus spurred by its representation in popular discourse as a response to disastrous social and political upheavals in sending countries (Hoffman 2012; Marre and Briggs 2009, 12–13).

International adoption is in fact but one end of a spectrum of activities that qualifies as an industry built around orphan rescue—from donations to organizations that target orphans to the establishment of orphanages and orphan tourism, international adoption, and even proselytization about international adoption. The orphan industrial complex is premised on a discourse of orphan rescue precipitated by the idea of an "orphan crisis," described in part 1, that traveled from development to charitable responses, all with dire consequences for child protection. Though it never really came to pass, the notion of an ongoing "orphan crisis" has persisted and spread beyond the professional development community to be commonly used by charitable organizations. In particular, the notion of an "orphan crisis" has been appropriated by the US evangelical community as a justification for widespread congregational encouragement to internationally adopt (Joyce 2013a). Arguing that the Bible commands Christians to help widows and orphans, the evangelical community is fueling the misappropriation of the term *orphan* to promote a missionary agenda that can actually put children at risk of institutionalization and trafficking. More and more Western evangelicals are buying into the discourse of orphan rescue, calling on followers to adopt and serve in orphanages as a way to "minister" to millions of orphans around the world through a gospel-centered method called "orphanology."[2] The Christian Alliance for Orphans (CAFO) promotes an annual Orphan Sunday to "defend the cause of the fatherless" (following Isaiah 1:17). CAFO also holds an annual Orphan Summit, which in its own words "has become the national hub for what Christianity Today called, 'the burgeoning Christian orphan care movement.'"[3] Rather than questioning the definition of *orphan* or what constitutes an "orphan crisis," however, the summit—which caters mainly to prospective adoptive parents and US adoption agencies working worldwide—encourages adoption over family preservation. As alternative care consultant Mark Riley pointed out to me, "CAFO are still funded partially by adoption agencies, and adoption agencies need orphans. . . . And the easiest way to get orphans is to make sure that you can categorize as many children as possible as orphans."[4]

Other Christian organizations, such as 147 Million Orphans (the number drawn straight from UNICEF estimates based on the definition of an *orphan* as a child who has lost one parent and implying the number of "orphans" in need of "saving") heed the call by soliciting donations that will help "break the orphan crisis cycle."[5] The charity also raises funds for orphanage construction and maintenance, "serving trips" by young missionaries to feed children at various orphanages around the world, and families' adoption costs. One young missionary even started an Addicted to Orphans merchandise line, including rubber bracelets, to fund her 2012 mission trip to a Ugandan orphanage, so people could now advertise their obsession with orphans and adoption.[6]

In addition, many well-meaning Westerners hoping to ameliorate the circumstances of orphanhood have traveled to poor countries and established orphanages, which are often funded by both soliciting donations and charging foreign tourists to volunteer for several days, weeks, or months. Such orphan tourism has sparked what Chris Walker and Morgan Hartley (2013) call "The Orphan Industrial Complex," in which orphans and orphanages become tourist attractions that serve tourists' posthumanitarian desires for cultivation of the self in solidarity with the world's poorest and most vulnerable (Chouliaraki 2013). Despite appearing benign and altruistic, the Western demand for experiences with orphans in the Global South engages children in developing countries directly with international capital through an increasingly prevalent lay humanitarianism driven by a politics of compassion rather than a demand for social justice for children (Freidus and Ferguson 2013). In fact, these discourses of orphan rescue act as a justification for the commodification of orphans even as they reinscribe children as passive victims, rather than advocate for better child protection. While many orphan tourists coming from afar think they are offering children the love and attention they deserve, in reality they may be causing serious damage to individual children's development as well as broader child protection systems. Such damage occurs because the building of orphanages, especially in poor communities, attracts or even entraps children in these institutions, alienating them from their families and communities and stigmatizing them as the orphanage solidifies the identifying label of "orphan." Even for those children legitimately placed in institutional care, having many different volunteers stream through for short periods exposes the children to repeated abandonment, ultimately making it all the more challenging for them to form attachments to adult caregivers (Richter and Norman 2010). A small study of orphan tourism in Ghana found that children quickly formed and broke attachments as they "are used to constant arrivals and departures of volunteers, seem to get attached quickly, but are very conscious of the fact that there is a leaving date" (Voelkl 2012, 36). As a result, relationship formation is distorted—including anxious attachment and superficial relationships—for children exploited in this manner.

Encouraging international adoption thus drives a highly lucrative adoption market that unnecessarily institutionalizes children and even "manufactures" orphans for profit (Smolin 2010; Cheney 2014b). But the orphan industrial complex actually goes well beyond tourism and orphanage establishment to pushing toward adoption and even child trafficking. For this reason, the United Nations Children's Fund, originally United Nations International Children's Emergency Fund (UNICEF) has responded to the proadoption community's appropriation of its orphan estimates with concern; UNICEF has made qualifying statements in line with the Hague Convention on Intercountry Adoption that reemphasize community-based care over institutionalization and international adoption (UNICEF 2010), but doing so has only earned the organization pariah status among various adoption proponents who, while using their generous orphan statistics, also call UNICEF antiadoption and even antichild (Bartholet and Smolin 2012).

The proadoption lobby has also become powerful in the United States, which accounts for 47 percent of all international adoptions (Selman 2013b). In 2013, US Senator Mary Landrieu of Louisiana introduced the Children in Families First (CHIFF) bill, which unabashedly aimed to allocate federal resources "to strengthen intercountry adoption to the United States" (US Congress 2013). Premised on the idea that adoptable children are languishing in institutions while US families are waiting to adopt them, the bill ostensibly eliminates unnecessary bureaucratic barriers in order to help settle institutionalized children around the world in American families. Yet CHIFF's authors minimized recent adoption scandals and ignored how children end up in orphanages in the first place. Further, CHIFF implied that the United States could link aid to developing countries to adoption policy—a practice explicitly prohibited by the Hague Convention on Intercountry Adoption, to which the United States is a signatory. Though the bill garnered early support but did not ultimately pass, adoption lobbyists have attempted to institute other laws with similar provisions.

The Political Economy of Intercountry Adoption in Uganda

In Africa, the orphans who need "saving" are ostensibly those affected by war or AIDS—though as I have shown throughout this book, most children orphaned by war and AIDS in Uganda, at least, are absorbed into extended-family networks. Nevertheless, adoptions from Africa tripled between 2002 and 2012, despite a worldwide decline (African Child Policy Forum 2012). Ethiopia became the first African country to break into the top ten sending countries in 2004 with 1,527 intercountry adoptions (nearly twice that of 2003). This was due to no particular crisis; although Ethiopia has had its share of civil strife, chronic drought causing hunger and famine, and high

AIDS infection rates over the years, none of these factors was the driver of intercountry adoption there. In fact, no country has ever invited intercountry adoption per se; rather, adoption agencies looking for supplies of adoptable children seek out new sources. These sources often tend to be in poor countries with weak child protection systems. In Ethiopia, regulations were lax and decentralized, such that foreign adoption agencies found it easy to "do business" with individual orphanages and the courts (Bunkers, Rotabi and Mezmur 2012). By 2009, Ethiopia had surpassed second-place Russia in real numbers, with 4,564 intercountry adoptions. In 2011, only China was higher, with 4,418 intercountry adoptions to Ethiopia's 3,456—though these numbers represent 1.7 adoptions per 1,000 live births in Ethiopia versus 0.27 adoptions per 1,000 live births in China (Selman 2013a).

Following a familiar pattern previously established in Guatemala, Vietnam, Cambodia, and other sending countries, the adoption boom in Ethiopia quickly led to numerous allegations of corruption and child trafficking, until the Ethiopian government decided in 2012 to drastically reduce the number of adoptions. By then, the intercountry adoption community was already looking for new frontiers. Uganda was not initially seen as an ideal candidate, despite its supposed abundance of orphans: the Uganda Children Act of 1997 imposed a restrictive three-year residency requirement for foreign adoptive parents (Government of Uganda 1997). However, when the US Embassy issued a visa for a Ugandan child under the legal guardianship of US citizens in 2007, the intercountry adoption community discovered that applying for legal guardianship could act as a loophole that would allow them to take Ugandan children out of the country and then finalize adoption in their home countries, though technically legal guardianships are still under Ugandan courts' jurisdiction (Namubiru Mukasa 2013). Legal guardianship is explicitly designated as a temporary arrangement *not* to be used as a means to adopt, but due to legal precedent (and, many observers surmise, financial incentive), Ugandan courts continue to grant legal guardianship orders to foreigners, knowing full well that they intend to take the children out of Uganda and file for adoption in their home countries (Alternative Care for Children in Uganda 2014). According to the US State Department, only 311 Ugandan children were adopted by US citizens from 1999 to 2010, but in 2011 alone, 207 Ugandan children were adopted by US citizens (Schwarzschild 2013)—a 400 percent increase from 2010 (Alternative Care for Children in Uganda 2014). In 2012, 238 of 254 total Ugandan intercountry adoptions were to the United States (Australian InterCountry Adoption Network 2015)—95 percent of them, according to Riley, through the legal guardianship loophole.[7]

These numbers may still seem small, but at approximately forty thousand

US dollars per adoption, Ugandan institutions are now recognizing that international adoption is a highly lucrative business.[8] Thus, evidence is already pointing toward alarming irregularities, including recruitment and inducement of birth parents to relinquish children under false pretenses, "child laundering" through altering and forgery of records (Smolin 2010), and extortion of funds from prospective adoptive parents. Often led to believe that they are agreeing to an arrangement more akin to fostering or educational sponsorship with adoptive parents, guardians may unwittingly give up their parental rights without realizing that they may never see their children again.

The high-profile case of Stuart Bukenya is emblematic of the pattern of child trafficking into adoption. In May 2009, a relative approached four-year-old Stuart's parents on behalf of his employer, a lawyer whom he claimed connected poor children in Uganda with families in Europe and the United States for financial support. They agreed to be referred and were soon told that Stuart was chosen to go to the United States to be educated by a white, Christian, American family—the Hodges—under a legal guardianship arrangement. The parents were promised regular communication with Stuart and that he would return every two years until he completed his education and returned for good. Believing this to be a great opportunity, they cooperated in the entire process, which they had understood as temporary educational sponsorship rather than permanent adoption. The courts granted the Hodges legal guardianship, but once they were back in the United States, the Hodges immediately filed for adoption and changed Stuart's name to Silas Hodge. Stuart's parents in Uganda returned to the courts to ask how they could get their child back, only to find that they had no legal recourse because they had signed relinquishment papers (NTV Uganda 2013).

These practices violate several principles of the Hague Convention on Intercountry Adoption, including informed consent; a child's right to a name, family, and nationality; and the principle of subsidiarity, as well as the no initial contact rule. In addition, it commoditizes orphans to a whole new level and breaks up families while bypassing the structural issues that put poor families in a position to consider giving up their children in the first place. In doing so, these practices generate "orphans" specifically for the international adoption market, particularly by targeting the most desirable children (healthy infants) rather than children truly in need of families—including those already in institutions due to abandonment or the death of their parents. But Uganda has not signed the Hague Convention on Intercountry Adoption—and indeed did not even approach the Hague Conference about the possibility until 2012—so it could be some time before more safeguards to protect against adoption irregularities are put in place in Uganda.

In the meantime, child protection and alternative care specialists have tried to close the legal guardianship loophole by calling for a moratorium through amendments to the Children Act. But certain key figures—including the attorney general, Peter Nyombi, whose signature is needed for a proposed moratorium—have vested interests in keeping the adoption pipeline flowing (Namubiru Mukasa 2013).[9] The Netherlands halted adoptions from Uganda in 2012 due to evidence of corruption, but other Hague signatory nations continue to allow their citizens to adopt children from Uganda.

At the same time, lack of regulations (or ability to implement them) makes it easy for foreigners to set up orphanages in Uganda.[10] According to Riley, "There are a number of reasons why people would start an orphanage. One is, they actually care, but they just don't know what the right thing to do is. The second is money. It's become an easy way of making money in Uganda because people just love giving money to orphans. The third is ego . . . they can save orphans, and that makes them a hero. So it's colonization all over again."[11] However, the establishment of orphanages encourages abandonment, especially in poor communities, which sometimes consider orphanages a form of free boarding school (as orphanages are often painted in bright colors and cartoon characters, similar to nursery schools). Social workers I interviewed also reported that foreign donors have instructed them to fill their orphanages with children, abandoned or not, because it pleases their supporters. Such practices not only perpetuate child rescue narratives that fuel donations for the establishment and maintenance of orphanages but lead to unnecessary child institutionalization and even "manufacture" of orphans—sometimes explicitly for the purposes of intercountry adoption (Cheney and Rotabi 2014). Orphanages thus become a product of the adoption industry, rather than the reverse (Briggs 2012, 56).

The orphan industrial complex in Uganda is further fueled by other successful international campaigns drawing attention to hardships suffered by Ugandan children. Most notable of these is Invisible Children, a campaign (also run by young US evangelicals) to help children affected by the civil war in northern Uganda, though the organization was roundly criticized after the release of its video *Kony 2012* for distorting the facts about the insurgency (which had not in fact directly targeted northern Uganda since 2006). According to Riley, "The knock-on effect of the Invisible Children campaign is we've seen hundreds and hundreds of children institutionalized because other organizations have thought, 'Great! If we talk about the LRA and Kony and the war, that's a great way of raising funds!' So we now have organizations who've got children who have never been to the north of Uganda using Kony and the war in the north as a fundraising PR [public relations] exercise."[12]

An October 2012 op-ed piece in the national *Daily Monitor* newspaper calling for regulation of foreign adoption also refuted the story that war had led to the increase in adoptions: "Children from the Acholi sub region only contributed 9.6 per cent of the adoption total between 2002 and 2007. . . . All things considered, the essential motivating factor behind foreign adoptions seems to be money" (Agaba 2012).

The Political Economy of Abandonment, Institutionalization, and Adoption in Ugandan Context

It is important to note that Uganda has no significant history of institutional care. In 1992, after decades of civil war and at the height of the AIDS pandemic when 16 percent of Ugandan children had lost at least one parent, only 2,900 children were in institutional care (Williamson and Greenberg 2010, 7). In 2013, 14 percent of Uganda's 17.1 million children—or 2.43 million—had lost at least one parent to death. Of these children, 45.6 percent have lost their parent(s) to HIV/AIDS (Uganda Ministry of Gender, Labour and Social Development 2011, 4). Despite an "orphan crisis" threatening to overwhelm traditional extended-family care, about 90 percent of orphaned children are still cared for in their families and communities (Joint Learning Initiative on Children and HIV/AIDS 2009, 2).

These facts both problematize the very notion of "orphan" as a salient local category and fail to explain trends in institutionalization: by 2009, the number of children in institutions had skyrocketed to 40,000, and by 2013, it had jumped to 50,000 (Alternative Care for Children in Uganda 2014).[13] Meanwhile, the number of child care institutions increased from 212 in 2009 to more than 600 in 2012 (Riley 2012). By late 2013, Riley notes, the number had risen to more than 800.

These numbers are also disproportionate to what we know about child abandonment in Uganda. While it is difficult to find reliable numbers, child protection agencies estimate that a few hundred children are abandoned annually, about half in the capital city, Kampala. They are typically left at hospitals or in semipublic places such as bus depots or pit latrines. While research is also lacking on the actual reasons why parents abandon their children, much speculation rests on the mothers' circumstances and moral character, as they are typically assumed to be young or "loose" women who have given birth out of wedlock. The social workers I interviewed, however, indicated that where they were able to reunify abandoned children with their families, poverty punctuated by temporary crises tended to be an overriding consideration in abandonment (as well as an obstacle to reunification). They also surmised that child abandonment is increasing due to a breakdown in the extended-family structure that would otherwise support mothers and children. Social worker John Kasule, who has decades of experience working in babies' homes, told me:

> People are positing that the reason kids go into homes is poverty, and they'll be better tended in the homes. But in actuality they're making them—and their families—more vulnerable . . . In a country like Uganda, children are a source of support for the family. They enhance the support because their parents are poor but they get support of the children, and then they can prosper . . . as one unit. But now when you pull out those children from there . . . the support you are giving the children far away from [their parents], the families are not benefiting from it.[14]

Nevertheless, as orphanages spring up around the country, so do orphans to fill them. So though many people may assume that orphanages are being established to meet the increase in child abandonment, again, it is more likely the other way around.

OBSTACLES TO DOMESTIC ADOPTION

For children whose families cannot be traced,[15] adoption is one of a range of family-based alternatives to long-term institutionalization, which has been found to be damaging to children's development (UNICEF 2011; Dozier et al. 2012). On the one hand, given that Ugandans pride themselves on their strong extended-family care system and therefore tend to advocate for community-based care of orphans and other vulnerable children, it is surprising that they would hesitate to adopt abandoned children. On the other hand, most people who foster children informally do so only for their relatives or close friends because they tend to distinguish between the permeability of social kin relations and the impermeability of biological kin relations. Due to limited conceptions of adoption under customary law that take place only within the adopter's blood line, Trynie Davel claims that "adoption outside the African conception of children as belonging to or being affiliated to a particular family . . . would not make sense. In addition, it cuts across the African practice of ancestor worship. A child who is deprived of its roots would lose contact with the patrilineal ancestors" (2008, 270).

Ugandans' reservations about adoption similarly revolve around a moral economy of "blood" as an essential element in the formation of these kinship bonds. Noting, following Janet Carsten (2013, S146), that "the many possibilities that exist for inserting blood or other tissues into discourses which are politically or morally charged are suggestive of the capacities these bodily materials have for metaphorical extension," I therefore examine here how "blood" acts as a metaphor for the immutability of identity and belonging or exclusion in Ugandan society.

As explained in chapter 7, "blood" is mainly operationalized in Ugandan[16] moral economies of kinship through powerful beliefs that demonstrate its significance as a tie that binds children to their patrilineage—even when paternity is not clearly established. The Luganda proverb "Blood always finds its way home" implies that children estranged from their fathers' clans are instinctually pulled back through their shared substance/kinship. As a central idiom of relatedness, "blood" thus acts as a basis for rejecting adoption of institutionalized children. Further, "blood" is seen not only as the binder of kinship ties but also as the carrier of essential characteristics and diseases that may have been inherited from the deceased or abandoning parents of children potentially available for adoption.[17] Jini Roby and Stacey Shaw even claim that "in some African cultures the adoption of a child is believed to introduce alien spirits into the family" (2006, 202).[18] Ugandan prospective adoptive parents reported that, to discourage them from adopting, relatives and friends regularly said things like, "You can't adopt because you don't know that child's blood! What if his father was a murderer!? Then he could be a murderer, too!"

The child protection system is thus in a difficult position of having to pit moral discourses of innocent children needing adoption against the local moral economy of "blood." To adopt in such a context means to disinvest in powerful beliefs about blood as a substance that immutably binds biological kin. Though adoption can be complicated by the immutability of "blood," some people are willing to take the risk because of similar cultural emphasis on biological reproduction; infertility is one of the biggest motivating factors for prospective adoptive parents in Uganda. In a country with a high fertility rate, where having children is a central marker of adulthood for both men and women, adoption is considered an undesirable last resort. Women especially must fulfill their reproductive imperative by providing children for their husbands' patrilineages. Infertility is thus an extraordinary burden for Ugandan women. In fact, women will often try to adopt a child without their husbands' knowledge to obscure their (or their husbands') infertility. Kasule told me about one woman who had come to him the moment her husband had left on an extended business trip in hopes that she could adopt a baby before her husband returned and pass it off to him as his own child to which she had given birth. When Kasule told her it did not work that way, she pleaded with him, saying that if she did not have a child, her husband would leave her.

Adoption of unrelated children can also be seen as a threat to others' entitlements to family resources. Catherine Nganda, a babies' home director and adoptive parent, told me, "[Many Ugandans] will still find it noble and good that an American or a British comes and adopts a child; that is noble to them. But for you, a Ugandan . . . they see you already have your own family."[19] Relatives tend to object to adoption because bringing another child into a family threatens the inheritance of "blood relatives." Because inheritance is executed through the male line, boys in particular pose a threat to others' inheritance claims. Boys are therefore both abandoned more often and seen as less desirable adoptees than girls.

Kasule told me that by the time most Ugandans approached babies' homes to adopt, they had mostly already come to terms with issues about "blood." But even where they had come to accept adoption, the formality, bureaucracy, and cost of the lengthy legal process tended to put them off. "Ugandans wonder why they should be taken to that task," Kasule said. "They say, 'We have already given ourselves to the love and we are taking the child into our care. Why do we have to conform to the legal processes?'"[20] Kasule said that in 2009, it cost about fifteen hundred US dollars to adopt domestically, but thanks to several government and private initiatives, it now costs only about two hundred US dollars—and several organizations are trying to eliminate administrative fees altogether.

These changes and a vigorous public relations campaign called Ugandans Adopt led by Childs i Foundation (2013) have helped reduce some of the stigma associated with adoption. Yet myths still persist that Ugandans do not want to—and cannot afford to—adopt. Even babies' home social workers at alternative care workshops I attended in 2013 were shocked to hear that there are Ugandans willing to adopt; indeed, many had not even realized it was possible (though they were well aware that foreigners could adopt in Uganda). Others were amazed that it actually costs Ugandans next to nothing, as they had unnecessarily retained lawyers who charged four hundred to five hundred US dollars per adoption procedure. If these professionals—whose job it is to place children in adoption—are so ill informed, then how can the general public know? Kasule and Nganda agreed that much more publicity was needed.

AFTER ADOPTION

Even after following through with a formal adoption, there were several important reasons why people who had adopted preferred to claim their adopted children as blood relatives. Vitale Mukasa's decision, which opened this chapter, had mainly to do with Mukasa's managing of his own relatives.

Claiming patrilineal descent for his adopted child reduced several burdens: relatives' claims on his resources, pressure to foster their children, and relatives' concerns about him bringing "bad blood" into the family.

As a middle-class Ugandan, Mukasa was motivated in part by avoiding family's claims on his wealth: "Relatives who are struggling might ask, 'Why didn't you take my child to raise!?'" he said. "If you want to stay in peace," you avoid taking on relative dependents.[21] In fact, most Ugandan adoptive parents I talked with had first tried informally fostering extended-family relatives before opting for adoption, but they had found it unsatisfactory for various reasons: it opened them up to criticism by the child's biological parents for the way they were raising the children, and biological parents could come for their children at any time, regardless of the bond the foster parents had forged with the children. As a result, they never felt that they could fully bond with the children for whom they cared. "I wanted somebody who I feel is mine," Mukasa said, and he felt he could achieve that feeling through adoption. Relatives would accept the girl if they believed she was his biological daughter, even if it meant he had had her out of wedlock. In fact, it was seen as honorable that he claimed paternity. But because acknowledgement by the patrilineage is still an important factor for adopted children, Mukasa and his wife told only his father—whose responsibility it was to give the child a clan name—that they were adopting the girl. Mukasa said his wife even agreed to the "official" story that the girl was the product of her husband's extramarital affair because, after all, "It's what she grew up seeing: her father would bring a kid from an extramarital affair, and they would be happy. It's normal! . . . And the women feel happy if you bring a kid into the home, rather than sending help for when the kid is outside. Because the mother would be calling [and saying], 'the kid is sick; he wants school fees' and then she is not sure of what you do when you go back. Maybe you are adding on a second kid. So she's happy if you stay and bring the kid in. That's the way it works."[22]

By contrast, Nganda, who openly adopted a son after having twin daughters, said, "Even now, many families will accept it, but some families . . . still don't recognize your adopted child the way they recognize your biological children . . . [and think that] they are not obligated to welcome that child into their lives." In sum, as Nganda notes, "Fostering is seen as noble, adoption as shameful."[23] Despite the cultural ethos that "it takes a village" and the liberal use of kin terms to describe carers far removed from nuclear family, fostered children are never really "yours"; their reciprocal obligations will always be to their biological parents. Caring for kin is seen as a generous act toward family and community—just as having children is seen as contributing to your family and community—but adoption is considered "cheating" on those obligations, and this incorporation of children from different "blood" could have disastrous consequences for the cohesion of the family unit.

Though Signe Howell has suggested that children who are abandoned in Africa become "non-persons" because their disconnection from "blood" lines means they "fall outside kinship" (2006, 189), Ugandan abandoned children are not considered "less human" than other children; on the contrary, regular media stories about abandoned children invoke vociferous outcry and much sympathy for the children precisely because abandonment confounds the dominant ethos of family and community care (hence the abandoning parent becomes pathologized). Rather, the issue is that these children's families and communities are *unknown*. Or rather, other families do not immediately adopt them because *they are known to be kin of another* and therefore could never truly integrate. Further, it is not necessarily the things that are discoverable by testing blood, such as HIV status, that put Ugandans off adopting children.[24] Blood contains certain "truths," but testing cannot discern the intangible qualities carried in blood that make adoption so risky to Ugandans. Indeed, tests are to some extent unnecessary; the child's prognosis is already written in blood's cultural scripts.

Kin Making as International Politics: Who Should Care?

Many anthropologists have challenged conventional biological definitions of kin by describing the way care defines relatedness in various cultures (Alber 2004; Weismantel 1995). Where "blood"-based conceptions of kin pose obstacles for domestic adoption in Uganda, the question of care as kin making is what drives debates about intercountry adoption. Though adoption can be viewed as a personally shameful acknowledgement of the failure to reproduce, opening to intercountry adoption is also sometimes seen as shameful on a national level: a failure of the nation to take care of its own (Dubinsky 2010).

The arrival of intercountry adoption in Uganda has thus spurred competition among various moral economies of local and international orphan care, particularly who gets to be family for which Ugandan children. Even while many Ugandans found the idea of domestic adoption unpalatable, they could be deeply suspicious of foreigners adopting Uganda children. Resistance to international adoption is based to some extent in colonial history, yielding concerns with contemporary trafficking and even slavery. Sometimes they were concerned with the potential for exploitation of Ugandan children, but other times they were concerned with children's rights to culture and identity. In a clash of kinship concepts and the geopolitics of child care, then, parental fitness becomes an international issue. Foreign adoptive parents, who typically come from wealthy Western countries, will claim they can give children from poor countries "a better life"—and birth parents relinquishing children often agree: "With the poverty level in Uganda," says Nganda, "there are so many parents who are willing to give up their children for adoption because they feel 'I have suffered. If my child is going to have a better life, why not?'"[25] Even Ugandan courts are making foreign adoption rulings on the premise that children will inevitably have "a better life" in a wealthy Western nation than they will in Uganda (Namubiru Mukasa 2013). Such moral self-discrimination among Ugandans themselves indicates an internalization of broader Western discourses of parental fitness based on both class and race (Briggs 2012, 87). In each case, the definitions of *best interests* and *a better life* hinge overwhelmingly on immediate material considerations—though many believe that other considerations, including long-term psychological health and belonging, should be equally important. Kasule told me, "When Ugandan families do foster or adopt . . . [children] are going to live within the same environment and sometimes are not all that well off except that [parents] are going to provide the love and bring up these children within the Ugandan community. So these children will not see themselves as strangers anywhere, whereas if they are adopted internationally, at times they get racial discrimination."[26]

However, adoption debates premised on who is better suited to give children "a better life" often miss the point: it is not a question of whether (overwhelmingly white) adoptive parents from the United States or Europe *could* raise children of color from abroad but why and how certain parents, communities, and countries lose them to begin with (Briggs 2012, 7). The "better life" discourse is thus used to mask the hegemony of an intercountry adoption industry that operates on inequality (Cheney 2014b), and the right to family is used to justify intercountry adoption by anyone who wants children (Howell 2009, 157–58). However, adoption advocates rarely invoke the right to family for impoverished birth parents and their children in sending countries. The right to family, it should be noted, is not the same as entitlement to parenthood, particularly at the expense of others' rights to family—not least a child's right to be cared for by his or her parents or a child's right to identity, nationality, and culture (United Nations 1989).

In a country where more than 50 percent of the population lives below the poverty line, being poor is not considered a legitimate legal or moral reason to relinquish one's parental rights. Kasule once asked me rhetorically, "What measures do you have in place that the poverty of a family not able to take care of a child is this?"[27] He set an imaginary bar with his hand. Kasule and many other child protection professionals thus urge the government to prioritize poverty reduction and increased family support to prevent child abandonment. There are in fact many such programs, but they are up against a powerful and moneyed intercountry adoption industry.

Efforts to promote domestic adoption also suffer as a result of material interpretations of the term *best interests* because they justify institutions with intercountry adoption programs favoring foreign adoptive parents over local ones. Nganda has seen it often, including when she began her own adoption journey. "I went to one adoption office at a babies' home," she said, "but the treatment they gave me as a Ugandan trying to adopt was different from what they gave an American, a white." She said she and her husband persevered despite apparent discrimination, but on top of all the negativity around adoption of unrelated children, such treatment could quickly put off other Ugandan prospective adopters. "It's that perception in Uganda many times that . . . whenever you see a white person, you automatically think 'money.' When you see a fellow black, you think 'broke,'" Nganda said.[28] By late 2013, thirty-five Ugandan adoptive families who were preapproved for adoption by the pilot Alternative Care Panel had been waiting for nearly two years to be matched with a child, while during that same period, hundreds of children went abroad with foreign adoptive parents.[29]

The opinions of adoptees are also conspicuously absent in these debates. While it is too early to tell how children of Ugandan origin are faring in foreign adoptions, studies of other adult adoptees show that, even where they feel well integrated in their families and communities, they often experience a loss of connection with their country of origin that is difficult to recover (Quiroz 2012; Yngvesson 2010). This sense of loss is especially true of adoptees whose adoptions took place under suspicious circumstances. As one Ethiopian adoptee to the United States whose adoption was marred by irregularities put it, "I missed nine years of growing with my family. I missed speaking my mother's tongue. I missed my friends and my culture. I missed the sounds and the smells and the bustle of my hometown. I missed everything. . . . Adoption didn't help me; it helped the adoption business. Adoption didn't 'save' me; it served the American view of adoption. Adoption didn't find families for me; it found me for families that wanted to look like heroes in their community and their churches. I wasn't saved from Ethiopia; I had Ethiopia stolen from me" (Lemma 2014).

Riley thinks it will not be long before Ugandan adoptees will be returning to ask tough questions: "I keep telling people in Uganda who are processing international adoptions, 'This will come back to bite them in the ass. Listen to what adoptees who have grown up are saying!' And they're going to come up short in Uganda. Pro-ICA [intercountry adoption] folks will say these cases [of corruption] are the exception, but they're already becoming quite common in Uganda, and the wave isn't even full on yet."[30]

Confronting Ugandan Moral and Political Economies of "Blood," Belonging, and Child Protection

Attention to the various moral and political economies of adoption has prompted Ugandans to reconsider their attitudes toward adoption, both in policy and in practice. Part of the reason the Ugandan government established a three-year waiting period for adoption was that it needed to be able to monitor the progress of a child in his or her new family, and it could not practically do so after the child left the country. According to Kasule, the government also wanted whoever parented Ugandan children to keep those children in touch with their cultural heritage. The presumption was that foreigners who stayed in the country for three years would have some familiarity with and appreciation for Ugandan culture. Under these circumstances, Ugandans speak less of "blood" to inevitably pull adoptees back, but cultural heritage is still seen as an integral part of a child's identity, so keeping children who were adopted abroad connected to Uganda is locally considered a marker of a responsible adoptive parent.

While some Ugandans see intercountry adoption as a unique opportunity, especially for children who might otherwise spend their childhood in an orphanage, the potential loss of heritage is still seen as a difficult trade-off with the better standard of living adopted children are likely to encounter in the Global North. It also raises concerns about exploitation and even some jealousy. Nganda said, "There are people you talk to and [they] say Ugandan children are going out, and yet you will find Ugandans fighting to go abroad themselves, so there is a conflict of interest. People want to go abroad because there are 'greener pastures;' it's a better life out there. But just as many are saying that the children should stay in Uganda because out there they are going to exploit them."[31]

The way that intercountry adoption has developed in Uganda, with scandals like the Stuart Bukenya case becoming more common, is not helping to raise locals' opinions of it. Because of noticeable increases in foreign adoptions and media attention to such cases, Nganda says, "[Ugandans] no longer look at it as noble. . . . They are now becoming more and more suspicious."[32]

Rumors have circulated that Ugandan children are being adopted abroad for purposes of slavery or organ harvesting, or even that they are being thrown off the Empire State Building.

Ugandan attitudes about domestic adoption and "blood" are still slow to change, but with more media attention to both international and domestic adoption, people are opening up to the idea. Nganda says that, due to recent government pilot programs and awareness campaigns, more Ugandans are considering formal fostering as a first step. However, analysis of adoption discourse in the local media suggests that there is still need to demystify the practice, and the primacy of biological reproduction in building families remains largely unchallenged.

The "Rescuers": Cogs in the Wheel of Child Protection

At the same time, many organizations promote international adoption as solution to the "orphan crisis," often without noting its inefficiency (high amounts of resources to "rescue" few children), its politics (how did children become orphans in the first place, and *who* is entitled to parent *which* children), or supporting local efforts to improve child protection. According to Riley, the idea of raising money to help a particular well-meaning Western family adopt one particular African child is far more popular among evangelicals than providing funding to build an entire child protection system in an African country. As shown, their actions can actually put orphans and other vulnerable children at further risk. As with earlier development interventions, the current evangelical orphan movement is concentrated on the "orphan" demographic to the detriment of other children with even greater vulnerabilities. Although they are generous, evangelical "orphan addicts" tend to direct funding toward orphanages and international adoption when in fact, according to child protection specialists, these interventions should have the least funding. Because of this discrepancy, Kasule notes that a pattern of intergenerational orphanhood is emerging in Uganda: children raised in orphanages are now having children and also placing them in orphanages.

Some concerned individuals are trying to challenge the underlying assumptions that are endangering the development of stronger child protection measures, but real change cannot come until donors, particularly those in the evangelical movement, understand the dynamics of orphan care on the ground. While some faith-based organizations are doing excellent work in child protection and family reunification, others are at the forefront of child institutionalization and thus disruption of the establishment of an effective child protection system. As Riley notes,

Almost 100 percent of orphanages in Uganda are funded by some kind of church or faith-based organization, faith-motivated and faith-driven—which tells you that people of faith care passionately about impoverished and vulnerable children . . . [but] the truth is, if you have the tough conversation about the damage of supporting and building orphanages and international adoptions being a huge part of the solution—and that it shouldn't be—it actually puts them in a place where they are not the heroes. They are actually a cog in the wheel of a wider child protection system . . . rather than being the ones driving and pushing and being the heroes of the situation. And that's tough for people's egos; that's tough for people to hear.[33]

However, Riley and many others in child protection in Uganda keep pushing for change. As Riley puts it, "we need to challenge this, because until this develops into something appropriate—and I'm pretty sure it can, but it needs to be led differently—then . . . whatever we do here is going to always be trumped by the money that comes from [the evangelical movement] . . . sadly, because we just don't have the strength in the systems here to be able to withstand a barrage of do-gooders who are doing the wrong thing."[34] Thus, more charitable donors need to question their motives and actions concerning "orphan rescue," based on empirical evidence from people working in child protection.

*

Anthropological studies of kinship have been predicated on the immutability of kin relations as expressed through a distinctly Western idiom of "blood," while non-Western cultures tend to practice more mutable forms of kinship (Carsten 2011; Howell 2006, 2009). Whereas, according to Carsten, anthropological studies of blood as substance have "highlighted processes of change and transferability in kinship" (2011, 19), they can also highlight immutability: the belief that, as with an incurable disease, one cannot change essential moral qualities carried in the blood. However, my discussions with Ugandans about orphan care indicate that while it may be acceptable for Westerners to adopt unrelated children from Uganda, Ugandans themselves must first overcome the immutability of "blood" and the primacy of biological reproduction if the society is to widely accept domestic adoption.

At present, however, the moral and political economies of adoption are pressing Ugandans to change their thinking about kinship and belonging to more mutable forms for the sake of keeping Ugandan children in Uganda. This change means that while the Ugandan moral economy of "blood" limits the social group of the family as immutably and exclusionarily bounded for adopted children, Ugandans are still able to claim abandoned children as "ours"—as bounded by the nation-state—and therefore entitled to remain in the country of their birth. "Blood" gets implicated in debates about belonging, but belonging is also a political debate, about children as resources (and burdens) in families and nations. Who should get to care for them determines which country they contribute to if their potential is realized.

As this book has demonstrated, even Ugandan children who lose both parents are not seen as "orphans" by their communities, whose members have a tradition of taking care of them. It is thus egregiously erroneous to equate a child who has lost his or her parents with a child who is without family and is therefore internationally adoptable. Yet such a way of thinking is what is happening in international adoption discourses, where adoption proponents and self-appointed child "rescuers" are misusing the same UNICEF definitions of an *orphan* as a child who has lost one or both parents to conflate children who are parentless with children who are adoptable (Bartholet and Smolin 2012). Under these terms, almost every child in our study would be adoptable, though they may be in households where they are being well cared for, albeit by guardians and caregivers who struggle to provide for them. Defaulting to adoption as a solution to orphanhood ignores this fact and does little in the long run to alleviate their suffering. It even stigmatizes poverty and justifies taking children from the poor to give to the rich. Most aid organizations still hold that building the capacity of caregivers to support and provide for orphaned children improves circumstances for entire communities in ways that removing individual children from families to put on the intercountry adoption market will not, but the organizations promoting community-based alternative care are often "outmoneyed" by the private donations of child "rescuers" and potential adoptive parents willing to pay as much as forty thousand US dollars to adopt a child. Indeed, many international adoptions in Uganda have involved taking a child out of one family in Uganda and placing them in another abroad. There is therefore need for careful regulation as the international adoption market encroaches on children's and families' rights in Uganda.

In the meantime, a number of organizations in Uganda are trying to encourage family planning, domestic adoption and formal foster care arrangements to ensure that the few children who are abandoned each year do not languish in babies' homes, where they can experience developmental delays. Sensitization campaigns through radio, television, and print media such as Ugandans Adopt are making some headway toward this end. Yet this attempted change in the perception of domestic adoption involves challenging the major stereotypes about "blood" and the bureaucratic obstacles. As a caller in to a Ugandan talk show about domestic adoption put it, "I think in Uganda most people are not so convinced with the idea of adopting other people's kids, and this is a mentality we need to change. We always adopt people who are our relatives and we are not willing to welcome outsiders to our homes. But we forget that these are kids, and they have hearts, and they need to be nurtured and to be loved. If we change that, a lot could really change for our country." Christine Sempebwa, an adoptive parent on the show, replied, "She is right; we need to change this attitude in our people in Uganda. We need to take care of ourselves, take care of our children. They are *all* our children, and the more of us who take on a child *here,* the better our children will be and the better our future of our country will be" (Childs i Foundation 2013).

PART FIVE

Conclusion

9

HIV/AIDS Policy, "Orphan Addiction," and the Next Generation

Children should be the first to benefit from our successes in defeating HIV, and the last to suffer from our failures.

ANTHONY LAKE, Executive Director, UNICEF (UNICEF 2014)

I think the ARVs [antiretrovirals] have shaped the attitude of young people my age, in a way that most of them got hope, mostly for those that have HIV-positive relatives . . . they have hope that the relatives will live longer than the expected time. It has created happiness in families. Because of ARV treatment, you find that most people are not sad about their parents being HIV positive . . . They can take care of the HIV-positive people easily without thinking otherwise. It has also helped us to take care of ourselves since we know how people suffer taking them.

SUMAYIYA, youth research assistant, 2015

Young people my age enjoy life more than they could twenty years ago. Positive and negative status does not matter much in a youth's life now. We are so associative and free to even share status. Personally, I have a friend who is on ARV treatment, and my sister who is positive with three children. I have no worry that AIDS will kill them one day for I know once there was no treatment, but now they are always healthy and it's my responsibility to remind them to take the drugs.

JAMES, youth research assistant, 2015

The narrative arc of this book spans approximately eight years, from when the youth research assistants (RAs) and I began fieldwork in 2007 to the conclusion of the writing in 2015. Even within this time, we have seen the evolution of policy responses to AIDS orphanhood from a practice of reifying orphans, to integrating them into broader policy, to actually creating orphans by separating children from family by drawing them into institutions, all in the name of "orphan rescue." As the quotes above from a couple of the youth RAs involved in this study indicate, however, they are aware that they are growing up in a different world than that of their parents due to the development of life-prolonging antiretrovirals (ARVs). Many of those who have been orphaned may no longer be crying for their elders but rather reciprocally caring for them, urging them to take their ARVs. Despite this welcome shift, the contents of this book have illustrated that orphanhood continues to be constructed in ways that misidentify or even obscure the true causes of orphan suffering—often with adverse, long-term consequences.

Gains and Losses in the Fight against HIV/AIDS

A number of recent developments continue to challenge the lives and liveli-hoods of the post-ARV generation. First, Uganda's HIV prevalence rate has begun to rise again, after years of steady reduction, and young people have some of the highest new infection and lowest ARV coverage rates. According to the 2011 Uganda National HIV Indicator Survey, the prevalence rate among Ugandans between fifteen and nineteen years old was 7.3 percent (8.3 percent among young women), up from 6.4 percent in the 2004–5 survey (Uganda Ministry of Health and ICF International 2012, 12). This increase is partly due to the enrollment of people living with HIV/AIDS in life-prolonging ARV treatment programs, but also because—despite a dramatic drop in the num-ber of new infections among children primarily due to successful prevention of mother-to-child transmission—adult rates of new infections remain high: new infections among adults even rose from 129,133 in 2010 to 139,178 in 2012 before dropping slightly again in 2013 to 131,279 (Uganda AIDS Commission 2014). Some observers suggest that this consistently high rate is because the greater availability of ARV treatments has transformed an AIDS diagnosis from a death sentence to a "lifestyle" change, creating a general complacency or even "AIDS fatigue" that leads to a resurgence of "risky" behavior. But UNICEF reports that AIDS-related deaths for adolescents aged ten to nineteen years old are increasing, despite a global reduction in AIDS-related deaths of almost 40 percent between 2005 and 2013 for all age groups (UNICEF 2014).

Some of the youth RAs confirmed this ambivalence when I recently asked them how they and their friends felt about HIV/AIDS now. Sumayiya said, "People of my age, some know that HIV/AIDS is a killer disease, and they try as much to prevent themselves from getting infected. Some of them, they don't care about HIV/AIDS. They think that ARVs will help them live longer. As I was growing up, kids knew that AIDS is a killer disease and they hated it, since it took their parents' lives." James added, "I think the availability of HIV treatment (ARVs) has changed people's attitudes in a way that it is a no-fear matter. Young people now take HIV/AIDS for granted since there is availability of drugs one can sustain on for long without signs and symptoms showing up. Now, it's not like in those days when treatment was clueless and one could hide from the public when infected for signs and symptoms could show up in a short time." However, he also detected some ambivalence in his generation's relationship to HIV/AIDS and ARV treatment: "Though it is a no-fear matter, a number of young people fear going for the HIV/AIDS test. Some take themselves to be sick already, waiting for signs and symptoms as proof of their status, and [then] seek treatment [rather] than starting drugs after a simple test."

Although many young people in the post-ARV generation may have "no fear" of AIDS, there may still be cause for them to worry. Although the Barack Obama administration initially pledged to reform the US President's Emergency Plan for AIDS Relief (PEPFAR) on coming into office, the program remains much the same as it was under the George W. Bush administration. Despite various international organizations such as the Joint United Nations Programme on HIV/AIDS (UNAIDS) and the United Nations Children's Fund, originally the United Nations International Children's Emergency Fund (UNICEF) pledging to create an "AIDS-Free Generation," the Obama administration gradually defunded PEPFAR over the 2012, 2013, and 2014 fiscal years (Aziz 2013). Critics of AIDS prevention policy are now attributing the rise in HIV prevalence to such American policy decisions and other failures in AIDS education, including comprehensive sexuality education in general (UNICEF 2014). This gradual defunding poses a major problem for Uganda and other African nations but most especially for children orphaned by HIV/AIDS, who are more likely to become vulnerable to HIV infection themselves, not because of transmission in the womb from their parents but from structural and social risk factors (UNICEF 2006, 21). AIDS is in fact the leading cause of death of African adolescents (UNICEF 2014). UNICEF and UNAIDS estimate that 110,000 Ugandan adolescents ages ten to nineteen were living with HIV in 2013, while 6,500 adolescents had died from AIDS the same year (UNICEF and UNAIDS 2016). This estimate is especially problematic when many young people—as with all of the HIV-positive children in our study—do not know their own HIV status (UNICEF 2014).

In response to these glaring exceptions in the fight against HIV/AIDS, UNAIDS and UNICEF launched the "All In to End Adolescent AIDS" initiative in February 2015. With the support of the United Nations Population Fund, originally the United Nations Fund for Population Activities (UNFPA); the World Health Organization (WHO); PEPFAR; the Global Fund to Fight AIDS, Tuberculosis and Malaria; the MTV Staying Alive Foundation; and various youth movements, "All In" intends to provide "a new platform for action to drive better results for adolescents by encouraging strategic changes in policy and engaging more young people in the effort" (UNAIDS 2015). According to UNAIDS, "*All In* focuses on four key action areas: engaging, mobilizing and empowering adolescents as leaders and actors of social change; improving data collection to better inform programming; encouraging innovative approaches to reach adolescents with essential HIV services adapted to their needs; and placing adolescent HIV firmly on political agendas to spur concrete action and mobilize resources" (UNAIDS 2015).

Although the "All In" initiative shows promise for reversing these worrying epidemiological trends by involving more young people directly in the effort, it remains to be seen to what extent it will lead to concrete gains, either in HIV reduction among adolescents or greater youth participation in such initiatives. It is unclear, for example, what role essential support such as comprehensive sexuality education will play in "All In" initiatives, despite the vast majority of adolescents becoming infected through sexual transmission. Further, "All In" pledges to engage young people, but with "All In" calling on "national leaders to coordinate, support and lead assessments of existing programmes and expand partnerships for innovation between the public and private sectors,"[1] young people's participation may once again be easily hijacked or usurped by others' interests.

Aside from inadequate policies posing a challenge to orphan survival, there has been no shortage of critics of AIDS prevention programming who have taken issue more generally with the entire notion of "behavior change." Robert Thornton's incisive ethnography, *Unimagined Community*, attributes behavior change discourses to a failure of imagination: "Significant change in HIV prevalence is property of the social network rather than of individual behaviour. We must redirect our attention, then, from the scale of the in-dividual—behaviour, psychology, risk assessment, and so on—to the scale of the social" (Thornton 2008, 55). While policy makers tried to claim that abstinence was a main component of Uganda's initial success in reversing HIV prevalence rates, Thornton argued that "the change in Uganda was a systemic change that involved synergies between behavioural and social changes, on the one hand, and change in the configuration of the sexual net-work, on the other. To neglect this is to nullify the potential for success in other countries. . . . The apparent simplicity of ABC [Abstinence, Be faithful, use Condoms] message, then, is an illusion" (Thornton 2008, 86–87). Despite the advent of ARVs, this illusion threatens to condemn the current genera-tion of orphans now reaching adulthood to an HIV/AIDS epidemic similar to the one that claimed the lives of their parents: according to "All In," only about 36 percent of Ugandan adolescents currently have "comprehensive, correct knowledge of HIV."[2] If these modi operandi are not changed, they will have disastrous consequences—not only for African orphans but also for the fight against AIDS itself. Numerous advocacy groups have therefore rejected abstinence-only prevention programs, calling instead for comprehensive sexuality education that emphasizes sexual and reproductive health and rights over ideological claims about individual behavior, noting that young people cannot be expected to make healthy sexual decisions when they are denied adequate information to do so. In 2015, a judge in California even ruled that abstinence-only sex education is in fact not sex education at all but a denial of young people's right to information (Culp-Ressler 2015). Efforts to offer more realistic comprehensive sexuality education face opposition from increasingly powerful faith-based groups that have been emboldened by PEPFAR's disproportionate emphasis on abstinence-only programming, but having spent 1.4 billion US dollars on abstinence programming since 2004, research has shown it to be totally ineffective at reducing HIV infection, age of sexual debut, or teenage pregnancies.[3]

The fight against HIV/AIDS clearly needs young people, and young people need to take a greater place in research and policy making. To do so, they need support to receive—and even redesign—comprehensive sexuality education and other capacity-building measures to help them make the most of participatory opportunities and to lessen the impact of HIV/AIDS on their own lives.

Overcoming "Orphan Addiction": Building Better Professional Child Protection Systems

Despite the fact that, as I have argued in this volume, the "orphan crisis" was largely averted by community-based care, it is still a powerful rhetorical tool for supporting certain interventions over others. Though structural factors are affecting children more than orphanhood per se, this powerful narrative still pervades charitable responses to AIDS orphanhood in Africa. But not only is it failing to alleviate conditions of orphanhood, it is even generating orphans where they do not exist. Instead, we need to focus on strengthening community and overcoming "orphan addiction."

Increasingly, child protection advocates are calling for ethical and appropriate alternative care systems that make every effort to keep children within kin care where possible and that provide a family-like care environment where kin care is not possible. Establishment of such care systems requires being attendant to a child's natural resource system as well as the wider context; that is, supporting families and communities in a manner that is economically and socially relevant to local systems and culture. For example, in Uganda, ethical approaches to child care include a concerted effort to identify the misuse of the term *orphan* and combat the proliferation of residential care institutions in a country with a strong history of family and community engagement in responding to the needs of vulnerable children (Alternative Care for Children in Uganda 2016). Such an effort in turn necessitates an army of professional social workers specialized in dealing with children. As of 2015, certified social workers are generally lacking in Uganda, and although the Uganda Ministry of Gender, Labour and Social Development has been trying to recruit qualified district-level probation and social welfare officers who are responsible for enforcing child protection, only 40 percent of the positions were filled—mostly with people unqualified to work with vulnerable children.

Workforce training has commenced, underscoring the importance of family preservation, including means and methods consistent with best practices in social casework. Deinstitutionalizing children is now a policy goal in many impoverished countries (Williamson and Greenberg 2010), but in Uganda, such efforts are up against an aggressive orphan industry that posits its institutions as good places for children—particularly for parents and guardians who see in them the opportunity to provide a decent education to their children at no cost to themselves (Riley 2014).

In 2015, amendments to the Children Act were proposed that would strengthen adoption law by closing the legal guardianship loophole, as well as other provisions to protect children such as the abolition of the death penalty for children and corporal punishment in all settings.[4] Though a coalition of unscrupulous international adoption agencies and other beneficiaries of the orphan industrial complex, such as former attorney general Peter Nyombi, lobbied against it, Parliament approved the amendments in March 2016 and sent them on to the President for his assent. Adoption agencies and Nyombi continued lobbying against it, but children's rights advocates counter-lobbied for the passage of the amendments.[5] President Museveni signed the revised Children Act into law in May 2016.

The Ugandan Child Rights NGO Network (UCRNN), a coalition of nongovernmental organizations (NGOs) focused on children's issues, has called for the establishment of an independent National Council for Children to replace the body of the same name that is currently housed in the Ministry of Gender, Labour and Social Development. The National Council for Children was meant to monitor the ministry's activities in relation to children, but as one UCRNN member put it, it is "a sleeping giant" that has been ineffective because the ministry's mandate already covers too much, and, as another UCRNN member put it, "the child cannot tell the parent what to do when the child still lives in the parent's house."[6] If, however, an independent National Council for Children were embedded in the new Children Act, it would lend children's issues more political clout and pave the way for the professionalization of child care. The Children Act amendments approved by Parliament in March 2016 include the establishment of such an independent body responsible for ensuring compliance to the Children Act, policy formulation, planning and implementation of child well-being policy, but again, the proponents of the act face political opposition from vested interests, some of whom have been profiting off of the suffering of Ugandan children and their families.

The lives and livelihoods of this generation of Ugandan children hang in the balance of local and international policy and politics based on problematic constructions of orphanhood. Though too many observers consider children's issues to be a side note to HIV/AIDS policy and humanitarian practice, Laura Suski has rightly claimed that

> humanitarianism cannot be meaningfully understood without addressing its relationship to childhood as a space where the tensions between dependency and empowerment are managed and mismanaged. The "humane" task, then, is not to idealize childhood as a space of innocence and to engage in a project largely aimed at its global export. . . . Rather, the task is to deepen the narrative of childhood suffering and the moral response it inspires. This requires attention to the experience and voices of children. . . . A deepened narrative of childhood also requires attention to the voice and experiences of families and adults in the Global South (Suski 2009, 218–19).

An effective way to achieve better attention to children's concerns is to provide for the meaningful participation of children and youth in research, practice, and policy. The youth RAs involved in collecting much of the ethnographic data on children for this book were themselves children affected by AIDS—the eldest in the post-ARV generation—and their insights into children's experiences of orphanhood in the age of HIV/AIDS have helped create not only a more incisive account of children's lives but a more precise picture of the (in)effectiveness of current interventions for children that can inform how we respond to children's actual rather than perceived vulnerabilities. Put simply, children are the experts on childhood. If we are to understand the politics of childhood, we need to continue to pave the way for young people's substantive involvement in research and policy making.

Acknowledgments

I would like to express my gratitude to the many people who saw me through this book.

First and foremost, I have to thank the children and families whose stories comprise so much of this book, as well as others who lent their insights and expertise. I could not have done it, however, without a fantastic research group: youth research assistants, known by the pseudonyms James, Jill, Malik, Michael, and Sumayiya. You are all very special to me, and this project is yours as much as mine. I appreciate the risks you took in engaging in very personal journeys through this research, and I'm so glad it helped you learn about yourselves as well as engendered compassion for others. I am most especially grateful to Faridah Ddamulira for her contributions to the project's success. Even today, you continue to "coordinate" my visits to Uganda and facilitate my continued contact with the children and families described in this book.

I appreciate numerous colleagues' constructive comments on many earlier formulations of this project at all the conference and workshop presentations of this work since it began in 2007. I especially thank the members of the ISS Children and Youth Studies writing group in The Hague—Auma Okwany, Roy Huijsmans, and Shanti George—for their careful readings and the insightful discussions they yielded. I am also indebted to the University of Chicago editors T. David Brent and Priya Nelson, who saw this book through a long development process. Finally, the anonymous readers provided invaluable feedback for the improvement of this volume, as did copy editor Lori Meek Schuldt and others at the University of Chicago Press involved in its production.

This project was financially supported by the Fulbright Africa Regional

Research Program (2008–9) and several University of Dayton Research Council Seed Grants (2007, 2008, 2009, 2010). Many of the chapters in this book were also redeveloped from earlier publications and are published with permission.

Last but not least, I would like to thank family, friends, and colleagues who either directly supported me or patiently put up with me during the prolonged writing process. Aside from my wonderful friends and colleagues in Uganda, I know Maarten Heesakkers has my back (with technical as well as moral support), as has Jessica Newman through many decades of friendship. My grandmother Mabel Rocamora was always my biggest cheerleader, though, and I regret that she did not live to hold this book in her hands. However, her spirit of inquiry and social justice imbues its pages.

Appendix

Children and Household Profiles by Youth Research Assistant Focus Group, 2007–2009

Youth Research Coordinator: Faridah Ddamulira
Youth Research Assistants (all of the following names are pseudonyms):

James (kindergarten): Belinda, Diana, Joel, Omar, Robin; Jaaja Hamidah's household
Michael (first grade): Darrin, Edwin, Jessie, Joanna; Marjorie's household
Malik (second grade): Wasswa, Kato, Carter; Jaaja Rose's household
Sumayiya (second grade): Barbara, Emily, Raj, Willy; Farzana's household
Jill (third grade): Norah, Pearl, Rose; Olivia's household

Youth RA James's Group: Kindergarten

BELINDA (GIRL): Belinda was a talkative, lively, and confident six-year-old girl who loved playing. But she could also get sick a lot and had a large rash on her body when we first met her. At the time, Belinda had tested positive for HIV, but another test in 2008 was negative. Belinda knew none of this. She lived with her mother's aunt, whom she called *jaaja* (grandmother). She drew her parents and siblings in her picture not because she lived with them but because she *wished* she did: her parents lived elsewhere while dealing with the effects of HIV/AIDS, and her twin older siblings were staying with their maternal grandmother. She also had a younger half sister who lived with her own father in a neighboring village.

Belinda indicated a strong relationship with her grandmother. She said that *jaaja* told her stories and sang to her as well as provided for her needs, but James observed a different story. Her *jaaja* had a tiny house, and Belinda was made to do some pretty difficult chores for a six-year-old. Belinda's *jaaja* supported the children by brewing homemade alcohol and selling it with roasted pork in a stall adjacent to their home. As the only child among adults (many of them her *jaaja*'s drunken customers), Belinda longed to stay with other children. She also feared that her *jaaja* would one day be eaten by a night dancer or wild dog because she at times dozed off without locking their front door—though James was concerned that it posed other dangers, under the circumstances. Her *jaaja*'s business often kept Belinda awake at night and made her late for school in the morning, where she would be punished for tardiness. James thought that Belinda seemed a bit more comfortable at school, maybe because she had a lot of friends and while at school she could forget her family problems. When James was doing activities with the group, Belinda was often the initiator.

Toward the end of 2007, however, Belinda's life changed. Her mother got very ill from AIDS symptoms and came to live with Belinda and her great-aunt. Belinda told James that her mother was always locked up in the house. Her mother had, in fact, run mad from illness, but no one was discussing the situation with Belinda; she was left to make what she would of her mother's erratic behavior until she died shortly thereafter. Belinda's father later died, and still Belinda was kept in the dark. According to James, Belinda was never the same after her father's death: she started keeping to herself, and even her *jaaja,* who was not typically concerned, got worried about her health. Belinda told James that she got to see her mother when she died, but she did not see her father, and she felt terrible that she did not get a chance to say good-bye to her father. However, she had pictures of both her parents and a *gomesi* traditional dress of her mother's that comforted her.

Belinda said her life would have been different if her parents were still alive. She felt that orphaned children suffered more than children whose parents were alive. She heard someone refer to her and her siblings as *mulekwa,* which to her meant "someone who belongs nowhere and is poor."

After a prolonged period of grieving, Belinda gradually reverted back to her usual self and became lively again. She even discussed her parents' deaths freely with James, which she previously could not do for at least a year. James took this willingness to talk to mean that she had come to terms with their deaths.

DIANA (GIRL): Diana was a painfully shy six-year-old girl who pursed her lips nearly the entire time we spoke to her and avoided being picked to participate in activities. We were not sure we would be able to draw her out, but her circumstances spoke to her demeanor: she had come to live with her paternal grandparents when her father died. Diana's mother remarried and moved far away. Within a few months of moving, her grandfather also died. Her mother never visited or called to check on Diana and her elder siblings.

In 2007, Diana was staying with her uncle and grandmother, though she identified the only other people in the picture that she drew as her mother and father, which was what she called her grandmother and uncle by then. Although she was not that close to them emotionally, she felt obliged to use familial terms, as they were her caregivers. She also lived with three cousins— two girls and a boy—but she told us she did not draw them in her picture because, she said, she did not like them; they teased her until her grandmother intervened. Her grandmother stayed around for six months after the death of her husband, but then she left the country to join her daughters in the United Kingdom, leaving Diana solely in her uncle's care. At the end of our first interview with Diana when we asked her if she wanted to add anything to what she had told us, she leaned close and whispered, "I would like to live in another place."

This comment seemed odd to us given that Diana's home was the nicest of her research cohort. At first, Diana's family did not welcome James because it seemed they had something to hide. With time, though, James learned the source of some of the tension in Diana's home: Diana's uncle was actually her father's stepbrother, so he did not feel he had much responsibility toward Diana. Though he was wealthy enough to have a big, fancy wall around the house's compound where he also ran a small paint factory and he sent his biological children to nice boarding schools, Diana was often left home with the maids to cook for the workers in her uncle's factory. She regularly missed school due to failure to pay fees.

This treatment made it clear to Diana that she was an orphan, and she felt as though orphans were treated differently from other children. It made her feel bad that her father was dead. She never talked about her mother. She once told James that her best friend was the dog, which later got hit by a speeding *boda-boda* (motorcycle taxi) and died a painful, slow death.

James observed that Diana felt uncomfortable around her uncle, who was worried that she would say bad things about him to James. She seemed to appreciate having a visitor check on her while home and always got sad when James would leave. We started becoming concerned for Diana, but then one of the maids contacted one of Diana's aunts, who took her in toward the end of 2008. Diana had to move homes again, but she got her wish not to live there anymore.

JOEL (BOY): In 2007, Joel was a reserved six-year-old who lived alone with his *great*-grandmother. His mother conceived him when she was fourteen years old, and then she left him with the grandmother who had been caring for her. The headmistress at Joel's school emphasized that Joel's great-grandmother is *very* old (which is a relative term, of course: I didn't get a number). He seemed to like it there because he even drew his neighbor playmate into his picture. His cousins were not far away, either, though they stayed elsewhere. He got to play a lot, but he also did some housework because his grandmother was so old: he washed dishes, collected firewood, washed clothes, and fetched water from the well. He actually liked sweeping the compound, unlike his other jobs. Every day when he got home after a long walk to and from school, he washed his uniform and dishes before playing.

Joel said his *jaaja* is kind to him, never yelling or beating him even when he has misbehaved. She told him stories, and though she was not able to afford toys and other luxuries, she provided his school supplies with help from an uncle, who later moved them both from a remote location closer to his home.

Joel did not know much about his mother aside from what his *jaaja* told him or the pictures she showed him. His mother got married, and though she was a teacher in Mbarara, she never visited Joel. He had no idea who his father was, either, but *jaaja* told James that Joel's father died in 2008 of AIDS. She tried to get in touch with his family so that Joel would get to know others in his clan, but they expressed no interest in Joel because he had been raised a Christian while they were Muslims. Further, Joel's father was married when he impregnated Joel's mother, so in order to save his marriage, Joel's father denied any involvement with the fourteen-year-old girl. Joel was thus not recognized among his father's relatives. Though he would have loved to live with his parents just like other children, Joel had known only his *jaaja* all his life and did not remember living anywhere else. He identified his biggest problem as the long journey (2.5 kilometers, or about 1.5 miles) that he had to walk from home to school every day, so all in all, he was doing fairly well.

OMAR (BOY): Omar drew his family in different sizes according to generation: his grandparents were biggest, his aunties and uncles were medium-size, and then his siblings and cousins were the smallest. In 2007, he was an inquisitive five-year-old who could easily be distracted and wander off. He stayed with his father's aunt near the school. He said his father lived somewhere far away, and he did not know who his mother was. His mother had died and his father was living with AIDS, often falling sick. His father's aunt said she brought him to live with her because no one was taking care of him in the village where he was staying with his father; he was not even studying. In fact, she was the one who raised Omar's father. She said he was really wild, dropped out of school, and got a lot of young girls pregnant—including Omar's mother. She confided at the time that Omar's father was refusing to take antiretrovirals (ARVs), substituting alcohol for them instead. Omar, however, talked to James about his father with much happiness, and it was obvious he was very fond of him. He sometimes visited Omar and brought him nice things like sweets and clothes. Though Omar had no memory of living with his parents and he loved living with his aunt, he sometimes wishes his father lived with them. Sometimes he would say that his parents were not staying with him like other parents who stayed with their children because they did not love him.

Omar was also very fond of his aunt and said she paid special attention to him, singing him songs and telling him stories. In turn, Omar helped out at home by going to the store to buy chicken feed and washing dishes. He did not share a bed with anyone, primarily because he wet the bed at night. Omar preferred home to school because he liked playing. He enjoyed building small houses and bridges out of clay, like his father, who was a builder. He said he wanted to be an architect.

Omar understood the term *mulekwa* as a child without a mother and a home. He went on to say that he was not a *mulekwa*, because he had a home (though he did not have a mother). He expressed that he would love to have a mother like other young children.

ROBIN (BOY): Robin's father died in an accident in early 2007, so I thought he might have some memory of his father, unlike some children who were too young when their parents died to really remember them. But in 2007, he appeared not to be aware that his father was dead; he thought that his father was staying somewhere with his mother. He missed them, but he said he did not cry about it.

Robin's mother remarried someone in western Uganda, where she also taught. He would go to visit her during holidays, but Robin and his older brother stayed with his maternal grandmother, whose husband died in 1982 in Uganda's civil war. She had nine children of her own, seven of whom still lived at home and were almost finished with school. Robin was the youngest child at home and was apparently adored by his aunts and uncles. His mother also sometimes visited him there.

Robin's mother decided to leave her children from her previous marriage with her mother because, first, she was sure her mother was the only person who could take good care of her children, and second, she did not want to cause any tension in her new marriage if her new husband did not acknowledge Robin and his brother.

Robin told us that he had a fairly big home with his own bed, a sign of relative affluence amid the children with which we were working. His house had electricity.

He loved to play on the balcony and watch television. He also did chores, though: he swept the compound and the kitchen, cleaned, fetched water from the well, and washed clothes. His grandmother sometimes went to Mbarara and left him with a neighbor.

Robin was a bit quiet but showed that he could engage in question-and-answer sessions. He also responded well to games and songs. Over the course of James's youth RA interviews with him, Robin showed he remembered his father and freely talked about him. He said that a reckless driver killed his father when he was thirty-one years old. He told James that when he grew up, he would not touch alcohol because a drunk driver killed his father. Robin was originally named Robert Junior, but he changed it to Robin, claiming that since his father was dead, he should not be using his name; otherwise, according to superstition, he could also die soon. Robin did not self-identify as an orphan, however.

Robin told James that life was good at his grandmother's house: he was never mistreated and had few chores. Being the youngest, most of the time he could play. All in all, however, he would love to stay with his mother if he could. His ideal family would comprise his grandmother, aunts, uncles, mother, father, and siblings.

JAAJA HAMIDAH'S HOUSEHOLD: In 2007, Jaaja (Grandma) Hamidah had lost three children, each of whom left her with two of their children. She lived with four of her grandchildren in a rented two-room apartment, while the two eldest were in boarding school. Their parents left them with her when they were young. The youngest was Justine, whom Hamidah knew was seven years old because her mother lived with Hamidah when Justine was born. "As such," Hamidah said, "I have watched her since she was a baby. My other grandchildren were brought to me after their fathers had died. Their mother would simply dump them at my home. In fact, some of them were dumped at my doorstep. So definitely, I just estimate their ages but I'm not really sure." She had no income but some money from selling charcoal, a business for which she had gotten a small setup loan. She had tried belonging to several women's finance associations, but she was too busy to attend meetings or did not find them helpful when she belonged to them.

Caring for so many children for whom she was not prepared took a physical and emotional toll on her, especially given that Justine and her older brother John were both HIV-positive. "Just looking at these innocent children suffering breaks my heart," she said. "Looking at and raising my grandchildren reminds me of my own dead children, which has greatly affected me emotionally."

John and Justine received free ARVs, but Hamidah struggled to even find money for transport to the hospital several times a week for checkups. She wished the organizations that provided ARVs would open satellite clinics in other areas so that they would have better access to health care for the children. She also knew they needed nutritious food, but she constantly struggled to provide for them. It made her feel like a failure.

Justine and John both died of AIDS-related pneumonia shortly after we met them (see chapter 6). Hamidah was so heartbroken at that time that the two other boys she cared for went to stay with other families while Hamidah moved to a different apartment to be away from the place where she had lost so many family members. Shortly afterward, the two oldest, one the elder sister of Justine and John, were short of school fees and so came to live with her.

Youth RA Michael's Group: First Grade

DARRIN (BOY): Darrin was a happy and lively seven-year-old in 2007. Though Darrin's parents were alive, they were HIV-positive and were unable to send him to school. He was living with his paternal grandfather when his aunt who sold street food at a secondary school canteen offered to take him and his brother in and enroll them in the community school assistance program. When Darrin had been in school for one year, he was bright enough to skip kindergarten and go to first grade with his age mates.

Darrin could sometimes be contrary. For example, when asked what he liked best at his home, he told us he loved the chairs. Later, he told us he hated sitting down while at home. He lived in a two-room apartment, and he shared a bed with his brother. He reported visiting his mother once, but he stayed with his grandparents during most holidays.

Toward the end of 2008, Darrin's aunt lost her job and also broke up with her husband. She could not afford her apartment thereafter, and so she moved to her village in central Uganda. We were not able to get a location of Darrin's new home and so lost touch with him.

EDWIN (BOY): Edwin was living with his father, stepmother, two older siblings, and younger brother in 2007. His older siblings shared a mother, but Edwin had a different mother and so did his younger brother. His parents quarreled all the time, and when they split, Edwin's mother left him with his father. When his father remarried, his new wife did not like Edwin and his older siblings, so she constantly mistreated them by denying them meals, clothes, and other essentials.

Later, Edwin's stepmother also separated from Edwin's father. Edwin and his siblings were left with their father and an aunt who came to help a bit as she searched for a job. They lived in a one-room apartment where Edwin shared a bed with his sibling. A small garden plot the neighbors let them use was one of their only food sources. His father was often ill and did not have enough money to feed them on a daily basis, so Edwin often came to school hungry and depended on school meals.

Edwin told us he did not have many friends around his home; most of them were at school. In fact, he told us he was not really allowed to play at home. He was responsible for many chores, including cleaning the house, sweeping the compound, feeding the pigs, fetching water, cooking, and washing. He got to play soccer with his friends at school, so he preferred it to home.

Edwin's paternal grandmother Jaaja Rose finally took pity on him and his siblings and took all the children into her already-crowded home. Edwin told his youth RA Michael that he loved it at Jaaja Rose's place. In fact, he said he loved it so much that he wouldn't want to live with either of his parents any-more: his mother constantly yelled and quarreled, and his stepmother constantly beat him while his father did nothing to stop it. His father was not physically bad to him, but he was either sick or never home, so Edwin was not close to his father at all. Edwin was also bitter that his father never helped them during those days when their stepmother mistreated them.

Edwin first struck us as a shy boy who spoke slowly, but when we got him into a focus group, he proved to be really sharp, catching on quickly to ideas. He was fidgety and energetic, and he would tell the research team grand stories. He developed a keen sense of justice as he got older and loved to talk politics. To him, a *mulekwa* was a child who was not treated well. He said he was a *mulekwa* while living with his parents and stepmother, but once he moved to his grandmother's house, he said, 'I am not *mulekwa* anymore because I am now treated well.'

JESSIE (GIRL): Jessie was a seven-year-old girl in the first grade in 2007. A double orphan who lived with her paternal grandmother, three sisters, and four cousins, she was a gregarious girl who smiled often. She also loved dogs, including her dog Snoop.

Jessie was well aware that her father had died before she was born. How-ever, at first she said her mother was alive and she occasionally went to visit her. We later learned that it was her aunt she referred to as her "mother." Her real mother also died when Jessie was young, and Jessie did not have the slightest idea who she was, nor did she have a picture or any memory of her parents. This lack hurt her, and she believed she suffered more than other children who still had their parents. She would have liked to know more about her parents, but she was afraid of asking her grandmother because her grandmother had made it clear that that was a closed chapter in her home.

Jessie's grandmother brewed and sold a local drink for income to take care of the children in her home. She rented her house and a small garden. Jessie initially lived with her aunt whom she called "mother" down the road in a mud-thatched hut, and she said she preferred living there because she had a lot of friends and few chores. With her grandmother, Jessie had many chores, such as gardening, which she did not like much even though that was their main food source. They also got some help from Jessie's employed paternal aunt, whose two daughters lived with Jessie at her grandmother's home.

She liked the people in her home, but Jessie also felt she was treated differently from the others; she thought her grandmother favored her living aunt's daughters more than all the other grandchildrens—perhaps because their mother is still alive and might be bringing special stuff for her own children. The research team noted that some grandparents tended to favor those children in their homes whose parents were still alive and provided some material support, unlike double orphans, who had nothing to offer. Jessie said she did more housework despite the fact that she was the youngest. Her cousins also had more clothes and shoes (Jessie had only one pair).

In 2009, Jessie's grandmother shifted to a faraway village after she was evicted from the place they were renting. She went with Jessie's older siblings, but Jessie was left behind with her paternal uncle, who lived a slight distance from Jessie's previous home. Jessie had no say in that decision and would in fact have wanted to move with her grandmother because she thought her uncle was rather stern. During holidays she could not wait to join her grandmother. She left her uncle's home immediately after the next school term ended.

JOANNA (GIRL): Joanna was an active seven-year-old who lived with her paternal grandmother, aunt, and cousins—two of whom were also in the same school. Two others went to a different school through sponsorship from an Australian. Her parents were both HIV-positive and separated, and her father was bedridden, so he chose to send her to his mother. All her life Joanna had known only her grandmother as a caregiver because she was brought to her while very young, but Joanna expressed that she would love to stay with her mother and father. When we asked Joanna where her mother stayed, she said, "On the phone," meaning she once called on her aunt's cell phone. She wished her mother would call more often. However, she was in touch with her father, a construction worker, and loved him very much. She even visited him in a nearby village. She knew that she could not stay with her father because he frequently fell sick, though she did not know what caused it.

Joanna's home was relatively nice, and despite her having to walk a long distance to school, we had assumed that she was doing well. Joanna did not feel that she was treated any differently from other children in her home, but her youth RA Michael observed otherwise: Joanna had no bedding, so she and an orphaned cousin piled their clothes together to make a bed that they shared every night. However, the other children whose parents contributed to her grandmother's household had proper bedding. Joanna did a number of chores at home, including cooking in turns with her cousins. She loved the flowers and a toy car she drew in her picture of home. She hoped to drive one day. She had more friends around her home, but she said she ate better food at school (rice and beans). Still, she loved her grandmother for taking care of her and providing meals. She also got along well with her cousins.

Joanna said she was not constantly bothered by it, but she would give anything to know who her mother was and would have loved to live with her. She wanted a mother to tell her stories and carry her when she was sick. Joanna had a dress that no longer fit her, but her father told her grandmother to keep it because Joanna's mother had brought it for Joanna when she was younger, so it was highly sentimental to her and all Joanna had of her mother. When her father died in 2008, she told youth RA Michael, "Nobody told me when my father died. I don't even have a picture of him."

Joanna once commented that she had seen their neighbors' children play the "orphan role" just to get material things. In fact, they got sponsorship for school fees from a church organization despite their guardians being relatively well off.

MARJORIE'S HOME: When I first went to visit Marjorie, a neighbor guided us to a house just behind the roadside shops that looked more like ruins. It was sitting out in the open, without a discernible compound boundary. The entire front half had been erected with bricks, but the floor, roof, and windows were missing. The erosion of the bricks, especially in the window frames, indicated that it had been sitting there for quite some time without being finished. In fact, an earthquake came along while we were in the house, and, given that I could even see light through the mortar in the brick walls, I was really tempted to bolt, worried that the house would come down around us (fig. 13).

We walked through to the back half, where they had covered the two back rooms with iron sheets. It was dark inside, and though they had furniture, the cushions were bare foam without covering. The cushions were rather filthy, too, and the household members covered the chair they wanted me to sit in with a shirt so I would not get dirty. It was apparent that they had little, and the kids were not that clean, either.

Marjorie, a slight woman in her mid-twenties (but who looked much older), had dropped out of university to care for her maternal aunt and her

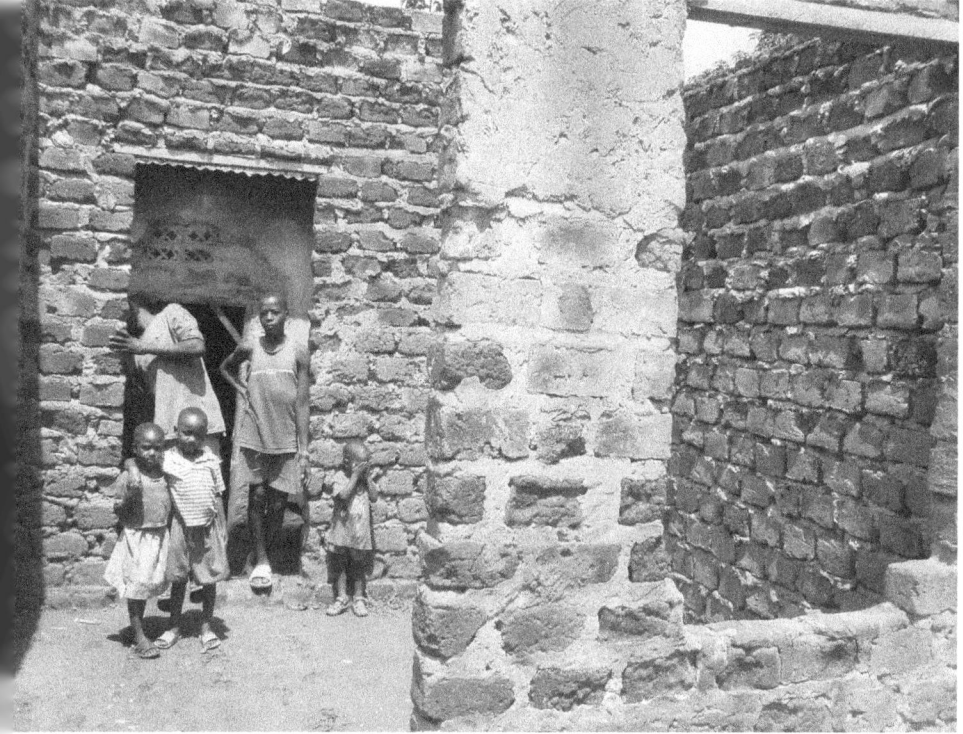

FIGURE 13. Marjorie's house in 2007. Everyone stayed in the back rooms behind these unfinished ones.

children. She cared for her aunt, who was dying, and her aunt asked her to continue caring for the children after she was gone. The house had initially belonged to Marjorie's uncle, who was given the land by an employer who had allowed him to start building on it. But when they had a conflict, the employer started selling off parcels of the land. The uncle tried to protest, but he was powerless to stop it. Then his wife died in 2002, and he passed away just two months later, before he could finish the house—leaving Marjorie as the head of the household. She stayed not only with the three boys of her aunt but also with her two young daughters and a sister to that aunt (fig. 14).

Marjorie suffered chronic health problems and could only get regular work as a local produce stand attendant, whose owner paid her 1,000 shillings (about 50 cents US) and a free lunch per day. She also did some laundry and gardening for people on the side.

As a result of their experiences, Marjorie and her charges were initially extremely morose, hopeless, and mistrustful of others. One could seemingly do nothing to get the two little girls, Aliya (age six) and Anna (age five), to smile, as both their fathers had abandoned them. When I asked what was

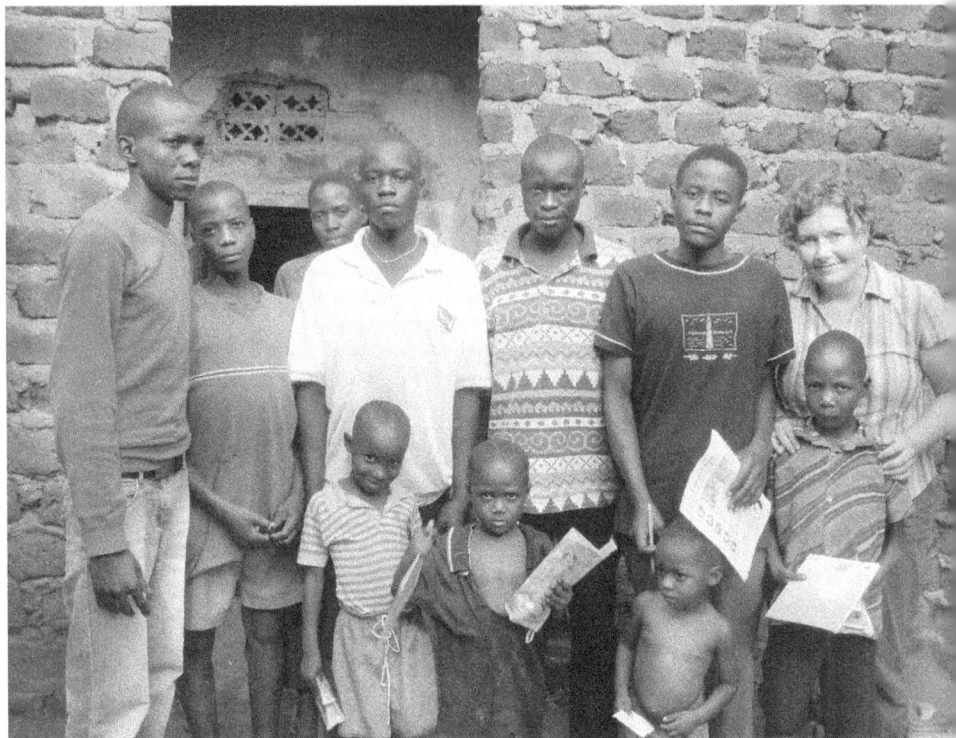

FIGURE 14. Youth research assistant Michael (*far left*) and the author (*far right*) with members of Marjorie's household.

new on a second visit, they all said, "Everything's the same," with resignation. "No one helps us," eldest brother Darren would repeatedly lament to youth RA Michael. Marjorie rarely engaged in conversations but looked on with her sad and defeated expression. It was fairly difficult for him to draw them out, but Michael solved that problem by coming with some of his old clothes and shoes, all of which fit one of the boys or another. Brian especially opened up to Michael, discussing his parents' deaths. He said he watched as his parents wasted away in pain during their long sickness. However, no one explained to the children what was wrong with their parents; they were constantly told that their mother had a fever, even while on her deathbed. They were not allowed to see her, so they never said good-bye to her. Before he could grasp the fact that he would never see his mother again, his father also died, and still no one offered an explanation. They were not allowed to discuss their parents in front of adults unless they were whispering. Brian suspected that both his parents had died of AIDS when he looked back at the way his parents had both wasted away with disease.

When asked what concerned them, Brian chimed in with "school fees." He had reason to worry, given that he was finishing primary school and wanted to go to secondary school so he could be a doctor or an engineer. He and the other boys worked weekends and holidays, doing odd jobs to raise their own fees. They were all concerned about the ability to stay in school, as it was the only thing that made them feel like regular children. They all said they preferred it to home. When I asked what they did not like about their home, Isaiah (age ten) responded, "I don't like the misery and sadness." Arthur (age seven) said, "I don't like the iron sheets [on the roof] because they leak when it rains." Brian (age fourteen) replied, "I don't like fighting or arguing with my brothers." They all agreed that their cousin Marjorie treated them well, though. The boys said their greatest wishes were "to be treated as kids, [to have people] help us with clothes and education, and to be treated like other children who have their parents . . . and to complete our house."

When the research team connected the family with a foundation that offered educational support, they were all smiles for the first time since we had met them.

Youth RA Malik's Group: Jaaja Rose's home

WASSWA (BOY): We met Wasswa when he was eight years old and in the second grade. He was the first-born of fraternal twins who lived with their paternal aunt, Rose. His mother did not get tested or tell anyone she had AIDS, so nobody knew why Wasswa was so sickly and slow throughout his infancy. When their mother died, Rose had both twins tested for HIV and it was discovered that Wasswa, who had been born naturally, was HIV-positive while his brother, Kato, who was born by cesarean section, tested negative. Rose had Wasswa enrolled in an HIV treatment program. He was one of three boys in the home on ARVs, but he and the others were unaware of their statuses. Wasswa in particular would tire of taking ARVs and constantly ask why he always had to take so many medicines. They would tell him it was because he had a "brain issue" that necessitated the medication.

Wasswa was playful and lively when we met him, and he actually looked healthier than his twin brother, who had a persistent rash on his face at the time. Wasswa knew little about his mother, and he missed his father, until he came to live with them. He felt well cared for by his aunt, though he would sometimes stay at school and avoid home to avoid taking medicine.

KATO (BOY): Kato was an energetic and sharp child who was protective of his twin brother, Wasswa. When Wasswa failed to take his medicine (sometimes on purpose), Kato would run back home and get it for him.

The twins had lived with their aunt Rose (whom they called *jaaja*, or grandmother, like everyone else) since they were toddlers. Their parents made the decision that Wasswa and Kato would stay with their aunt before they passed away, so since their infancy they had lived with their aunt. Their father came to live with them when he became bedridden with AIDS complications. However, the twins were not aware their father had AIDS; they thought he suffered from kidney failure and would be getting an operation— which was also partially true, as he had an inserted tube that helped him pass urine.

Kato did not remember his mother, who died when he was two years old, but he became frightened about their father's health and also became attentive and protective of him as well as his brother. He hoped to be a doctor one day.

CARTER (BOY): Like his twin cousins, Carter was eight years old and in second grade in 2007. He lived in the same household as the twins, with Jaaja Rose. He too was HIV-positive, though his younger sister was not. He was unaware of his HIV status, but he was curious and intelligent, and his aunt worried that he would find out. His mother had died in 2004, but his father was living with AIDS. His father sent Carter and his younger sister to their grandmother's after he became too weak to work, so Jaaja Rose provided everything for them, with the support of other relatives.

Carter was an emotional little boy with a keen sense of justice who could be sullen and reserved. He took everything he was told seriously and thought carefully before he spoke. He also stood his ground once he made up his mind about something. On one occasion at school when his teacher removed some of his break-time edibles from his food container, Carter refused to attend class until everything had been replaced. He also once refused to be punished for coming late to school because he had to do housework first thing in morning, unlike other children who only had housework after school.

Carter remembered little about his mother, but he gradually revealed some deep-seated anger toward his parents for leaving him and his sister with their grandmother. He was also rather upset with his mother for dying, as if she had a choice, and was similarly critical of his father for not taking better care of himself so that they could stay with him.

Though he could be hard to draw out, Carter sometimes expressed a desire to be included. In his drawing of things he liked, he drew only a two-story house, a truck, and a bicycle. He explained that life is great when you live in a beautiful two-story house and have a big car like a truck to enable one's whole family to move about. We later learned that on many occasions Carter and his young cousins had been left home as the elders went to parties due to lack of an adequate vehicle to ferry all of them at once. The bicycle was to enable him to get to school on time and also to run to the shops to help his grandmother pick up certain things.

JAAJA ROSE'S HOUSEHOLD: Jaaja (Grandma) Rose was taking care of fourteen of her grandchildren, nieces, and nephews (three of whom were HIV-positive and receiving ARVs) as a result of losing four of her eight adult children and some other relatives to HIV/AIDS. Three more of her children were seriously ill at the time, so only one of her children was alive and well. This brave woman was also taking care of her younger brother (father of the twins) and a son, both of whom were in the terminal stages of AIDS. She lived in an unfinished house and sold charcoal to feed the children. She was well regarded in the community, and some surviving relatives of the children and neighbors helped her with food.

The children in Jaaja Rose's house (including Shekinah and Travis, who were mentioned in chapter 4) seemed to get along well, and most of them who had lived there for a while called each other "siblings." As some of her daughters passed away, Jaaja Rose considered letting some of the children go to the fathers' families, since it was customarily supposed to be their responsibility (see chapter 7). But then she worried that perhaps they would be mistreated in those households, so she brought them to her house. Not only did the children not always know who was their sibling and who was their cousin, but Jaaja Rose often slipped between calling the children her grandchildren, nieces, or nephews and just referring to them all as her children (fig. 15).

Each of the children on ARVs had to go to receive regular checkups and medications at hospitals and clinics on different days because they each had different doctors. Sometimes an older sister to some of the children would go to pick them up and bring them, but the doctors recommended that if the children showed even the slightest sign of sickness, they should be brought in for a checkup. Since this happened fairly often, it meant that the children also missed school on those days.

On a visit in 2014, Faridah and I asked Jaaja Rose how many children she had fostered in her home over the years. She and her adult relatives started counting on all fingers. "Thirty-two or thirty-three," she concluded.

Youth RA Sumayiya's Group: Second Grade

BARBARA (GIRL): Barbara is Rwandan, and she and her two older sisters came to live with her paternal aunt in Uganda after her Rwandan father died when she was two years old. Her mother also died shortly afterward. She did not realize that her parents were dead because her aunt just told her they were

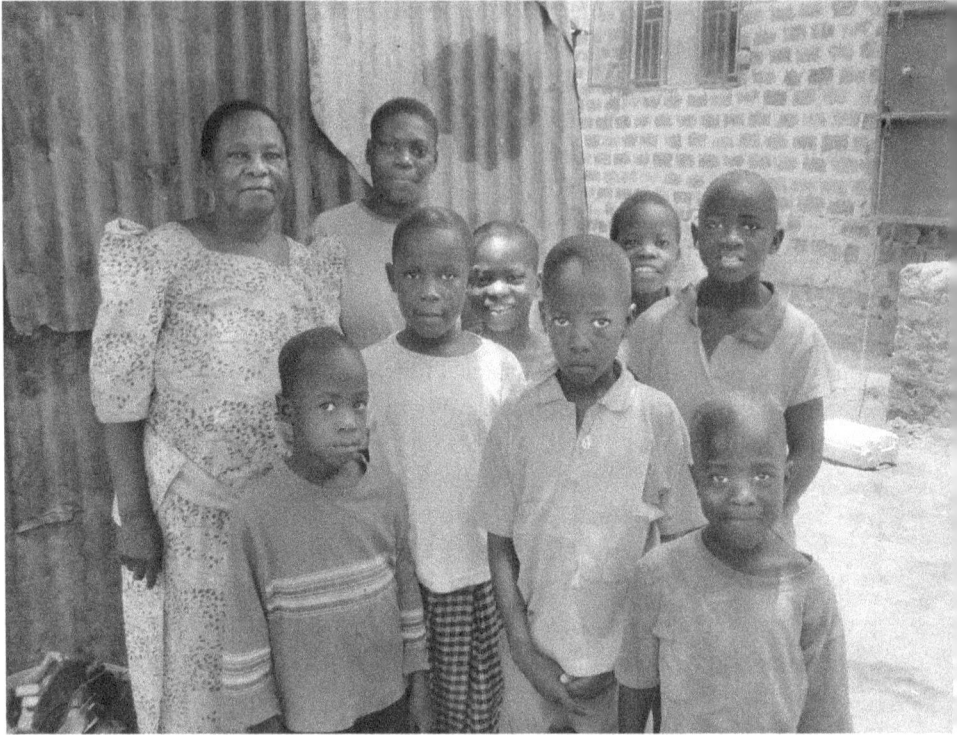

FIGURE 15. Jaaja Rose (*left*) with some of the children in her care, photographed behind her house in 2009.

in Rwanda. Once in a while, Barbara would express discontent at the fact that her parents never communicated with her and wondered why they could not just call to say hello, or she could never go for holidays in Rwanda to be with her parents. She was just told that it was too expensive and far away. She told us that her favorite game was called "Mother and Father," a game of pretend modeling the nuclear family.

Barbara clearly felt different in her home. She constantly complained that she was made to do most of the chores. Her older siblings went to boarding schools on a church sponsorship, and during holidays they did all chores together with her, but while they were away, Barbara suffered a lot. Her aunt's children also lived at home, but they went to nice schools in Kampala and they were driven to school daily. However, Barbara had to walk to the community school every day.

In our initial interview, she was a bit shy and spoke softly. But when she was in the focus group sitting next to her friend Emily, she became really animated, even stubborn and opinionated. When we were describing what we do each day, I went first. I described my day and ended it with going to sleep. She expressed shock: "Don't you pray!?"

In 2008, Barbara stood her ground, saying she would not go back to school unless she was taken to a nice school in town like her sisters. One of her uncles found her sponsorship, and Barbara got her wish.

EMILY (GIRL): Emily loved school and wanted to be a teacher when she grew up. At eight years old, her parents were separated and she lived with her mother, maternal grandmother, elder sister, and brother. Her mother had no job but got some money for cultivating others' gardens as well as a small plot of their own. Emily did not know much about her father, who never contacted her—though her mother still had some pictures. As first, they lived at her maternal uncle's home, but Emily's grandmother asked her and her mother to move in with her after Emily's grandfather died. Her maternal uncle paid her and her siblings' school fees, so she was never out of school. Emily fetched water, washed dishes, and cleaned the house, but she felt loved and well supported there and did not want to live anywhere else.

Emily was a lively, playful girl who volunteered information freely. When we asked about her favorite game, Sweet Potato, she demonstrated the little song and dance that go along with it. During focus group discussions, she would whisper, giggle and joke with her friend Barbara.

Emily knew she was not an orphan, but she thought that some orphans led better lives than children whose parents were alive. For example, her friend Barbara got a sponsor in 2008 and went to a better school. She felt hurt when Barbara left, but they still saw each other at church on Sundays. She also felt the absence of her father as well as her deceased grandfather.

RAJ (BOY): Raj guessed that he was six years old, but like many children, he was not really sure of his age (and neither were many of their guardians, especially when children had no birth certificate). We thought that would be unlikely given that he was in second grade, but when you saw his diminutive size relative to his classmates and his quick wit, it might just have been possible.

He was aware that his father had died and his mother was sick with "fever." She stayed in a village in western Uganda. Raj stayed with a woman everyone thought was his grandmother, a nurse, and his aunt, though it later turned out that the supposed grandmother was just a friend to Raj's maternal grandmother, who lived in western Uganda with Raj's mother. During one of her visits, she asked Raj's real grandmother for Raj and Sharina [Raj's nine-year-old female cousin], promising to look after them and send them to school, since they were staying home during that time. However, she was actually looking for children to work in her home. Raj performed such tasks as washing dishes and clothes, cleaning the house and compound, and fetching water.

These chores often made him late for school, and his friends would tease him, though Raj would always smile and attribute his lateness to the long distance he walked to school. He also never carried any snacks for break time like other children. For that reason, Raj did not take mundane things for granted. When asked what he would do if given a lot of money, his first reaction was "school fees" and supplies including pencils, pens, and books. Later, he added that he would buy a plastic container to pack break-time snacks such as *mandazi* (fried bread) and *chapatti* (flat, unleavened bread). He also said he would use the imaginary money to buy transport to school.

Raj eventually confided to youth RA Sumayiya that he did not actually like it at the home of his "grandmother." In his old home in the village, he said, he was treated like a young child. When asked to clarify, he said, "Young children there do minimal work. When they fall sick, they are allowed to rest and not do housework. They are allowed to play. Young kids are not sent out to the shops at night; adults do it. And young kids are brought new clothes, especially on big days like Christmas." Raj also remembered how his mother used to sing him nice songs and play with him before she started falling sick. The last time he had seen his mother, she was crying and hugging him. He thought it was because the doctor had just given her an injection. Raj therefore feared injections.

After being tipped off by a neighbor who saw how much Raj and his cousin Sharina were being mistreated, the Local Council intervened, forcing the old lady to return Raj and Sharina back to their relatives. We lost touch with them after they returned to the West in 2008.

WILLY (BOY): Willy drew an incredibly neat picture of his home, complete with sugarcane in the foreground. At ten years old, he was talkative, intelligent, and informative, though he pointed out that he was not the best performer in school. He stayed with his paternal grandmother and younger sister. He told us that both of his parents were dead, though he did not know why or when they died. In fact, his mother had remarried after his father died, leaving him with his grandmother when he was quite young. She never contacted or visited him anymore, so she was as good as dead to him. His grandmother did some small-scale farming, and their uncle helped out once in a while. They still struggled and went without meals sometimes. He shared a bed with his sister and did most of the housework.

Willy cared deeply for his younger sister, and he worried about what would happen to them if their aging grandmother were no longer in a position to care for them. In 2008, his fears came true when his grandmother's health failed her: she could not walk due to pain in her legs and swollen arms, so she could not cultivate the garden, and they experienced food shortages.

Willy also ran into trouble at school when his truthfulness and sense of fairness threatened to expose the headmistress's corrupt claims to a foreign sponsor that she allowed many destitute children to go to school for free when in fact she did not. She even started spreading rumors that Willy was a thief and chased him from the school, so he switched schools in 2008.

FARZANA'S HOUSEHOLD: Farzana was seventeen years old and was the head of her household, raising her three younger siblings (fig. 16) and a niece—two boys and two girls—ages five to thirteen years old (including Zack—see chapter 6). Her mother died when she was young (she did not remember the year), and her father passed away from AIDS in 2001 without arranging care for his children. Her older brother lived nearby with his wife and child in a one-bedroom apartment, so he looked after them, but their house was too small for all of them. Farzana's family lived in a two-room house in poor condition; it had a dirt floor and no windows, and the corrugated tin roof leaked whenever it rained. The elder brother drove a *boda-boda* (motorcycle taxi) and sometimes helped them with food. A paternal uncle, a maternal aunt, and even neighbors occasionally provided the household with

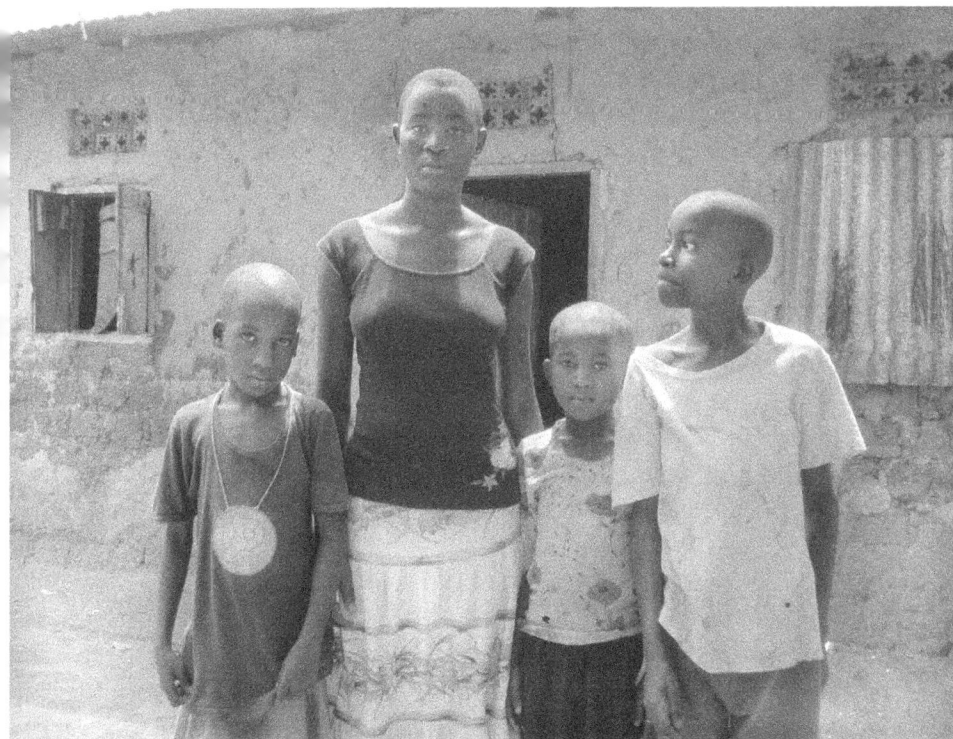

FIGURE 16. Farzana and her cousin (*left*) and two younger siblings in front of their house.

some basic necessities, but they could not provide regular school fees, so the children were out of school more than they were in school.

Farzana was in high school, and so when there was a lack of money, her fees were the priority in the hopes that she could finish and then find work to send the others to school. None of the younger children were in school in 2007. Being the head of the household was a challenge for Farzana in pursuing her education, however: "When they fall sick I at times have to miss school. There are times I leave school very tired; however, when I get home, I have to cook and do other housework. This really stresses me, especially during exam time when I have to read my books." She wanted to be a doctor.

Youth RA Jill's Group: Third Grade

NORAH (GIRL): Norah was a reserved eight-year-old girl whose initial drawing startled us because, aside from its apparent neatness, it was one of two in the whole school where the student included graves: she drew two graves in the *matooke* (plantain) garden and listed them as "my mother" and "my father."

Both of her parents had died by the time she was three. Her father died first, then her mother. She later tested HIV-positive herself, though the family did not disclose it to her. When we interviewed her, she pointed out that her parents were actually buried in their home village—not where she lives now—but since we had asked the children to draw their families, she decided to include them.

Norah's grandmother said the decision to stay with her grandchildren was made by her daughter before she died. Apparently her daughter conceived and gave birth to all her children while still living in her mother's house. In fact, she helped her deliver two of the children at home, so basically Norah had lived with her grandmother all her life. However, her grandmother was worried that her granddaughters were continuing the cycle: two of Norah's elder sisters had had children as teenagers while still living with her. The eldest sister had had two children by the time she was eighteen years old, and Norah's fourteen-year-old sister Agnes gave birth when she was thirteen years old.

Norah's grandmother did not work, although they got some food from a garden growing on land that had been loaned to them by the neighbors at the back of their house. They also had a cow that was given by one of the community organizations to households with kids living with HIV. They also got some assistance from her aunt and uncle who lived next door and were a relatively strong presence in her life. She did not get along well with her older sisters, however, who often assigned her heavy chores in the absence of her grandmother and uncle, perhaps because her grandmother tended to favor her. The others in the focus group joked with Norah that she was always the last one of them to arrive at school, but Norah said that she had to complete her chores at home, and the teachers beat her for it.

People in the neighborhood call Norah a *mulekwa*, and although she identifies with the term, it does not bother her. Her grandmother spoke openly and fondly of her parents and had some pictures of them, so she maintained a recollection of them. Norah told us she did not remember her parents very well, but she often went to weed her parents' graves, and it rarely upset her anymore because she was used to it. She had a keen sense that her life changed when they died, however; she said she fell sick more often, regularly getting "fever," a popular euphemism for HIV-related symptoms.

PEARL (GIRL): Pearl wrote sentences such as "I want TV" and "I want car" across her drawing, but she added, "I do have school fees."

Pearl told us she lived with her mother and stepfather in a rented one-bedroom apartment. Pearl indicated that her stepfather did not want to take care of her. It seemed that her mother was pressured to neglect her children: Pearl and her older sister Sandra slept together on the floor of a storeroom. Pearl felt that keenly: in the initial interview, she referred to her step-siblings (not drawn into her picture) as "Mother's kids" rather than as her siblings. Pearl, however, seemed fairly confident and well adjusted given her circumstances, which she may just have decided to accept. She never talked back, but she would ask, "Is it because I am an orphan? Is that why am I being punished innocently?"

Later, we learned that the woman she called her mother was in fact her maternal aunt Mary. Unbeknownst to Pearl, her biological mother had died when she was two and her father died when she was four years old. Mary told us that when Pearl's mother died, Pearl and Sandra were first left with their maternal grandmother. Two years later, though, their maternal grandmother also died, and their father, who was seriously ill at the time, took them in. A few months later, he also died, leaving them with his parents. One of their paternal aunts took them from the village to her home. However, the paternal aunt was mistreating the children, using them as servants in her home. So the maternal aunt went and convinced the paternal aunt to let her take them. She tried at one point to tell them that she was not their mother, but they got upset, so she dropped it and never brought it up again.

When Mary got married, she says life changed for Pearl and Sandra; her husband was not ready to take care of children that were not his. He did not even acknowledge Pearl and Sandra's presence in his home, and he took any opportunity he could to punish and mistreat them. He never let them touch the things he brought his children, and he never helped Mary with their school fees. Mary was torn between protecting Pearl and Sandra and her marriage. She felt guilty that she had removed these children from their paternal aunt because of mistreatment and here they were being mistreated in her home.

Neither of them had much to support the children, as Mary only had a small kiosk where she sold pancakes and vegetables and her husband was a fishmonger. When their home was broken into and her stock was stolen, as well as her husband's bicycle with which he delivered fish, she decided to contact another of Pearl's paternal aunts, who was headmistress in a certain school. In December 2008, Pearl and Sandra moved to their paternal aunt's home. They were actually happy there when Mary went to check on them. They told her about the nice things their aunt had brought them. They were excited to be going to boarding school. Pearl had to repeat fourth grade because she failed the fifth-grade interview, but she was still happier there. They planned to visit Mary during holidays.

ROSE (GIRL): Rose was another child from Jaaja Rose's home—her namesake, in fact. She was quiet, but she paid attention to our conversation, smiling a lot if saying little unless directly addressed. Her father died of AIDS in 2005, by which time she was already living with her paternal grandmother. Her mother was still alive in 2007 but went mad after her father's death and was bedridden with AIDS symptoms—a fact not necessarily known to Rose. She once told youth RA Jill that she had heard people talk about "this disease" (AIDS), and like other children, she perceived it as some sort of punishment for sinners who abandoned their families (children and wives). She had been at her grandmother's home for so long that she did not remember living else-where, yet she said she missed being with her parents, and she confided to Jill that sometimes she cried, though she hid her feelings from her grandmother. She fondly recalled being carried by her father before he died.

Rose was also fond of her elder brother David, who also lived with Jaaja Rose, and at times she confided in him. Like many of the children in the study, Rose found comfort in living with her siblings; much as she loved her cousins and other relatives, having her older brother there made her feel safer.

When we talked about how she spent a typical day, she said that she usually did not have any breakfast, and when she went home for lunch, her grandmother rarely had food, so she had "dry" tea (hot tea without milk) and popcorn.

Rose loved animals. Jill would sometimes visit to find her bathing the goat. Rose had some chores at home and liked to be at school, where she had many friends and enjoyed playing dodgeball. She hoped to become a teacher when she grew up.

OLIVIA'S HOUSEHOLD: Olivia was a university student who lived with her sister and her sister's children. Her sister, who farmed with her husband before he died of AIDS in 2002, also became ill, so Olivia brought her sister to her home and cared for her until she died in 2004. Before she died, her sister asked that Olivia keep the children together in her home. When she passed away in 2004, the rest of them stayed together in the same two-room house separated by sheets (see chapter 7).

Jacob and Agatha were both old enough to remember their parents well. They recalled fond memories of their parents providing nice things for them and playing with them. But everything changed after they died. Jacob was distinctly angry about his circumstances and did not like to recall how nice things were before because it only made him feel bad.

Olivia was studying to be a teacher. Apparently, a German man came around with a friend who lived in the area when Olivia's sister was still alive but bedridden. He took pity on them and offered her sponsorship. He did not sponsor the children, though, so to raise the fees, Olivia and the children helped cultivate neighbors' gardens for pay. At the end of the day, all four of them together might make 5,000 shillings (US $3). Olivia's grandmother also lived farther up the road, so they would get some of the food from her garden to bring home. Olivia also had a surviving brother who helped here and there, and eventually, she got Jacob and Hakim's paternal uncle to help with fees. When he went to Sudan on business, however, they lost touch with him, and all the children dropped out of school. By then, Olivia had finished her course, but she had not managed to find a teaching job. To make matters worse, part of their house collapsed in heavy rains. No one was hurt, but they had no money to rebuild it, so they all had to squeeze into one room of the house.

Notes

Introduction

1. In 2007, the number of orphans was estimated to be 2.2 million. By 2012, it had risen to 2.7 million (UNICEF 2013), but it did not double.

2. All names in this book are pseudonyms except for those of public figures.

3. Young Lives: An International Study of Childhood Poverty website, accessed April 4, 2016, http://www.younglives.org.uk/.

Chapter One

1. "Antiretroviral Coverage (% of People Living with HIV)," World Bank, accessed June 24, 2015, http://data.worldbank.org/indicator/SH.HIV.ARTC.ZS. This figure is 1 percent higher than the estimated 37 percent across all low- and middle-income countries.

2. This figure compares with 23 percent ART coverage of all HIV-positive children in low- and middle-income countries. These numbers fall far short of the 2015 Millennium Development goals (UNICEF 2014, 2).

3. He gave permission to tell his story anonymously.

4. PEPFAR Watch website, accessed July 24, 2013, http://www.pepfarwatch.org/the_issues/abstinence_and_fidelity/ (site discontinued).

5. "Uganda: 'Abstinence-Only' Programs Hijack AIDS Success Story: US-Sponsored HIV Strategy Threatens Youth," Human Rights Watch, March 30, 2005, https://www.hrw.org/news/2005/03/30/uganda-abstinence-only-programs-hijack-aids-success-story.

6. Viva staff in Kampala, interview with author, March 30, 2009.

7. "The President's Emergency Plan for AIDS Relief (PEPFAR) Blueprint: Creating an AIDS-Free Generation; Fact Sheet," US Department of State, November 29, 2012, http://www.state.gov/r/pa/prs/ps/2012/11/201195.htm. For the blueprint itself, see President's Emergency Plan for AIDS Relief 2012.

Chapter Two

1. Dorothy Oulanyah, interview with author, March 9, 2009.

2. The CRC's articles 20 and 21 deal with fosterage and adoption of any child "deprived of his or her family environment" (United Nations 1989).

3. John Okiror, interview with author, March 3, 2009.

4. Dorothy Oulanyah, interview with author, March 9, 2009.

5. Baker Waiswa, interview with author, March 4, 2009.

6. I have seen this happen in other instances where children find sponsors—particularly when placed in boarding schools.

7. Oulanyah, interview.

8. Foreign religious organizations are also implicated in highly controversial antihomosexuality legislation (Cheney 2012; Kaoma 2012) and orphan interventions that disrupt the development of an effective child protection system (Cheney and Rotabi 2014).

9. Sarah Kintu (UWESO), interview with author, April 14, 2009.

10. Viva staff, interview.

Chapter Three

1. There is a robust body of children's studies literature that takes on the issue of children's competence to act as rights bearers. The historical evolution of thinking about children's competencies and entitlements to rights bears striking resemblance to women's struggles for recognition of their humanity. Most scholars agree that age designations are somewhat arbitrary in determining children's competence.

2. I have had several editors of publications with which I was involved ask me to redirect my criticisms away from the actual text of the CRC and toward its interpretation and implementation instead.

3. Viva officers, interview with author, March 30, 2009.

4. Oulanyah, interview.

5. Auma Okwany, personal communication with author, 2013.

6. Okiror, interview.

7. Although Uganda has youth members of Parliament (MPs), *youth* are defined chronologically as any people ages eighteen through thirty-five. Youth MPs do not therefore advocate for children's interests but rather for those of young people in their twenties and thirties.

Chapter Four

1. Such interactivity can be considerably more difficult in societies such as the United States, where children are under greater adult supervision and surveillance to prevent abuse or abduction.

Chapter Five

1. The Ugandan Government only slightly altered this policy in 2009 through a directive from the Ministry of Education and Sports to allow pregnant girls in candidate classes to return to school and take their examinations (Ahikire and Madanda 2014, 2). For more on expulsion and reentry policies for pregnant students and young mothers, see Kamusiime and Okwany, forthcoming.

2. "Trafficking for Vulnerable Youth and Women in Kosovo," n.d., accessed April 13, 2016, http://www.pvptcenter.net/eng/Downloads/Trafficking%20prevention%20for%20vulnerable %20youth%20and%20women%20in%20Kosovo.doc.pdf.

3. "Malaysian Police Rescue 21 Ugandan Sex Slaves, 3 Other Ugandans Detained," *Washington Post*, accessed October 18, 2011, http://www.washingtonpost.com/world/asia-pacific/malaysian-police-rescue-21-ugandan-sex-slaves-3-other-ugandans-detained/2011/10/18/gIQATDfXtL_story.html (link no longer active).

4. Ugandan law defines *defilement* as sex with a girl under eighteen years old. Despite the crime carrying a maximum penalty of death, defilement remained a common occurrence. But few men who defile girls are actually convicted, usually managing to settle the dispute privately with the girls' families through a negotiated payment of reparations (Malinga 2010).

Chapter Six

1. *Dictionary.com*, s.v. "suffer," accessed April 14, 2016, http://dictionary.reference.com/browse/suffer?s=t.

2. Waiswa, interview.

3. These names are not pseudonyms, but since they are the names given to all twin boys—Wasswa is the firstborn and Kato the second born (whereas twin girls are called Babirye and Nakato, respectively)—they essentially conceal their identities as well as any pseudonym would, with the added benefit that they are ethnographically correct.

4. Though Indian generic ARVs were being imported earlier, they were limited to those who could afford them and were only made widely available and affordable in Uganda starting in 2004, with funding from the US Presidential Emergency Plan for AIDS Relief (PEPFAR), the World Bank, and the Global Fund, which negotiated to produce generic drugs that reduced individual treatment costs from US $1,500 to $30 per month (Whyte 2014; "African ARV Roll-Out," *Mail and Guardian*, June 16, 2004, http://mg.co.za/article/2004-06-16-african-arv-rollout). As with the twins' mother, however, many stigma-driven rumors and misconceptions made people reluctant to pursue treatment, even when it became more affordable and accessible.

5. This was early in the study, when we were recruiting families with which the youth RAs would work. As with other ethnographic anecdotes, the information shared here is thus a combination of my direct interaction with the children and their families and the reporting of the youth RA who worked with them from 2007 to 2009. In some cases, follow-up information gathered after 2009 by Faridah and me is also included.

6. "Uganda: Alarm as Uganda Moves to Criminalize HIV Transmission," All Africa, May 9, 2014, http://allafrica.com/stories/201405091564.html.

7. However, the World Health Organization determined in 2011 that "guidance for disclosure to children ages 12 and under constituted an unmet need and that disclosure to adolescents over 12 years required further and separate attention" (World Health Organization 2011, 17).

8. *Balekwa* is the plural form of *mulekwa*, meaning "orphan," but these terms do not connote the same kin relations as UNICEF's definition of *orphan*.

Chapter Seven

1. This type of decision making often leads to siblings being split into separate relatives' households, despite the fact that siblings are crucial sources of comfort just before and after a parent passes away (Kelly 2003, 73).

2. Each was born to a different father.

3. Alternately, this situation leaves girls who grow up outside their patrilineal clan less pro-

tected against sexual exploitation. Oleke and colleagues found that female orphans who lived with their mothers were frequently sexually abused, especially if their mother had remarried and they now lived with a stepfather's clan (Oleke et al. 2006, 277).

4. I have also heard from others that younger children are usually more desirable for labor because they are more easily manipulated and can be educated cheaply with the introduction of universal primary education (UPE) in 1997. Older children may also refuse to do work and start to make educational demands on their adoptive kin.

5. For a full explication of the term *mpisa*, see Cheney 2007b, 59–60.

Chapter Eight

1. Both names are pseudonyms.

2. Orphanology in the Authors' Own Words website, accessed April 29, 2015, http://www.orphanologybook.com (content no longer available).

3. "CAFO Summit," Christian Alliance for Orphans (CAFO), accessed April 21, 2016, http://www.christianalliancefororphans.org/summit/.

4. Mark Riley, interview with author, October 24, 2013.

5. "About Us," 147 Million Orphans, accessed April 21, 2016, http://147millionorphans.org/about-us/.

6. "Are You an Orphan Addict?" *Em on a Mission* (blog), December 6, 2012, http://emonamission.blogspot.com/2012/12/are-you-orphan-addict.html.

7. Riley, interview.

8. Ibid.

9. This statement is supported by personal communication in 2013–14 with a number of people who preferred not to be named. However, it was common knowledge that Nyombi was running a law firm that has been facilitating intercountry adoptions ("Foreigners exploiting law loophole to adopt, say MPs" *New Vision*, May 28, 2015, http://www.newvision.co.ug/new_vision/news/1327214/foreigners-exploiting-law-loophole-adopt-mps). In March 2015, Nyombi was ousted in a cabinet reshuffle, and there was renewed interest in passing the Children Act amendments that would close the legal guardianship loophole and lower the length of residency required to adopt. Nyombi was exceptionally vocal in opposition to the passage of the bill, writing paid "advertorials" in national newspapers defending his law firm against allegations of facilitating fraudulent adoptions (Nyombi 2016) and attacking the bill—even after Parliament approved it—as unconstitutional (Kasozi 2016).

10. According to Alternative Care for Children in Uganda (2014), only about thirty of the estimated eight hundred to nine hundred child care institutions currently operating in Uganda are licensed by the government.

11. Riley, interview.

12. Ibid.

13. It is important to note, however, that this figure does not represent the number of children abandoned in Uganda. An estimated 85 percent of children in institutional care have at least one living parent (Alternative Care Uganda, accessed April 2, 2015, http://www.alternative-care-uganda.org/current.html;content no longer available).

14. John Kasule, direct communication with author, October 23, 2013.

15. Most institutions have few or no funds for tracing families.

16. While conceptions of the role of "blood" vary slightly among ethnic groups in Uganda,

people I spoke with discussed "blood" as a general Ugandan concept, hence my discussion here reflects those conversations.

17. Such ideas predominated in Europe and North America until demographic shifts forced adoption into the international and interracial realm—and thus out of the closet (Dubinsky 2010, 10).

18. This notion is not limited to Africa or the Global South, either. Just reference popular American horror films for depictions of "demon adoptees" and "zombie birthmothers" (Nelson 2010).

There have also been numerous reports of evangelical Christian adoptive parents in the United States physically abusing adopted children as a means of expunging their "rebellious" ways that do not conform to strict fundamentalist codes of modesty and obedience (Joyce 2013b).

19. Catherine Nganda, telephone interview with author, December 12, 2013.

20. Kasule, direct communication with author, October 23, 2013.

21. Vitale Mukasa, direct communication with author, April 2, 2009.

22. Vitale Mukasa, interview with author, April 9, 2009.

23. Nganda, telephone interview.

24. By contrast, the files of many children being adopted internationally by Western adoptive parents will include blood tests to determine whether the child has any medical problems.

25. Nganda, telephone interview.

26. John Kasule, direct communication with author, November 5, 2013.

27. Ibid.

28. Nganda, telephone interview.

29. Riley, interview.

30. Ibid.

31. Nganda, telephone interview.

32. Ibid.

33. Riley, interview.

34. Ibid.

Chapter Nine

1. All In website, accessed August 3, 2015, http://allintoendadolescentaids.org.

2. Ibid.

3. "Promoting Abstinence, Fidelity for HIV Prevention Is Ineffective, Study Finds," *Medical Press*, May 2, 2016, http://medicalxpress.com/news/2016-05-abstinence-fidelity-hiv-ineffective.html.

4. On July 23, 2015, I attended a hearing in the Ugandan Parliament between the Gender Committee and the Uganda Child Rights NGO Network regarding proposed amendments to the Children Act.

5. Personal communication from several children's rights activists in Uganda who wished to remain anonymous, April 2016.

6. A public statement and personal communication, respectively, July 23, 2015.

References

Abdelmoneium, Azza Omerelfaroug Abdelaziz. 2008. *Non-Governmental Organizations and the Rights of Displaced Children in Sudan.* Institute of Gender Studies, Radboud University, Nijmegen, Netherlands.

Abebe, Tatek, and Asbjorn Aase. 2007. "Children, AIDS and the Politics of Orphan Care in Ethiopia: The Extended Family Revisited." *Social Science and Medicine* 64 (10): 2058–69.

African Child Policy Forum. 2012. *Africa: The New Frontier for Intercountry Adoption.* Addis Ababa: African Child Policy Forum.

Agaba, Marlon. 2012. "This Country Urgently Needs Strict Guidelines to Regulate Adoption." [Kampala, Uganda] *Daily Monitor,* October 1. http://www.monitor.co.ug/OpEd/Commentary/-/689364/1521464/-/l15vwl0z/-/index.html.

Ahikire, Josephine, and Aramanzan Madanda. 2014. "A Survey on Re-Entry of Pregnant Girls in Primary and Secondary Schools in Uganda." In *Survey Briefing,* edited by Maricar Garde. Kampala: UNICEF Uganda.

Alanen, Leena. 2001. "Explorations in Generational Analysis." In *Conceptualizing Child–Adult Relations,* edited by L. Alanen and B. Mayall, 11–22. New York: RoutledgeFalmer.

———. 2011. "Editorial: Critical Childhood Studies?" *Childhood* 18 (2):147–50. doi: 10.1177/0907568211404511.

Alber, Erdmute. 2004. "'The Real Parents Are the Foster Parents': Social Parenthood among the Baatombu in Northern Benin." In *Cross-Cultural Approaches to Adoption,* edited by Fiona Bowie, 33–47. New York: Routledge.

Alderson, Priscilla, and Virginia Morrow. 2011. *The Ethics of Research with Children and Young People.* London: Sage.

Alternative Care for Children in Uganda. 2014. "The Problem." Accessed January 2. http://www.alternative-care-uganda.org/problem.html.

———. 2016. *Strengthen African Families: The SAFe Campaign; A Call for Change.* Accessed April 22. http://www.alternative-care-uganda.org/resources/safe-campaign-brochure.pdf.

Aries, Philippe. 1962. *Centuries of Childhood.* London: Cape.

Arts, Karin. 2010. *Coming of Age in a World of Diversity? An Assessment of the UN Convention on the Rights of the Child.* The Hague, Netherlands: International Institute of Social Studies of Erasmus University.

Asad, Talal. 2003. *Formations of the Secular: Christianity, Islam, Modernity.* Stanford, CA: Stanford University Press.

Aspaas, H. R. 1999. "AIDS and Orphans in Uganda: Geographical and Gender Interpretations of Household Resources—Reconsidering the Domestic Mode of Production." *Social Science Journals* 36 (2): 201–26.

Australian InterCountry Adoption Network. 2015. "International Adoption Statistics." Accessed April 1. http://www.aican.org/statistics.php?region=0&type=birth.

Aziz, Rabita. 2013. "Obama 2014 Budget: Continued Support for Global Fund, Paired with PEPFAR Cut Leave Blueprint Goals in Question." Center for Global Health Policy. April 10. http://sciencespeaksblog.org/2013/04/10/cut-to-pepfar-support-for-global-fund-in-obama-2014-budget-leave-blueprint-goals-in-question/.

Barot, Sneha, and Susan A. Cohen. 2015. "The Global Gag Rule and Fights over Funding UNFPA: The Issues That Won't Go Away." In *Guttmacher Policy Review.* Washington, DC: Guttmacher Institute.

Bartholet, Elizabeth, and David Smolin. 2012. "The Debate." In *Intercountry Adoption: Policies, Practices, and Outcomes,* edited by Judith L. Gibbons and Karen Smith Rotabi, 233–54. Burlington, VT: Ashgate.

Bates, Robert H., V. Y. Mudimbe, and Jean O'Barr, eds. 1993. *Africa and the Disciplines: The Contributions of Research in Africa to the Social Sciences and Humanities.* Chicago: University of Chicago Press.

Bauman, Laurie J., and Stefan Germann. 2005. "Psychosocial Impact of the HIV/AIDS Epidemic on Children." In Foster, Levine, and Williamson, *A Generation at Risk,* 93–133.

Baxter, Jane. 2015. "The Archaeological Study of Children." Allegra Lab: Anthropology, Law, Art and World. May 12. http://allegralaboratory.net/the-archaeological-study-of-children/.

Bernal, Victoria, and Inderpal Grewal, eds. 2014. *Theorizing NGOs: States, Feminisms, and Neoliberalism.* Durham, NC: Duke University Press.

Bernard, Edwin J. 2014. "Uganda: Civil Society Coalition Condemns President Museveni for Signing HIV Prevention and Control Bill into Law." HIV Justice Network. August 20. http://www.hivjustice.net/news/ugandas-president-museveni-signs-hiv-prevention-and-control-bill-into-law-contradicting-evidence-and-human-rights/.

Bikaako-Kajura, Winnie, Emmanuel Luyirika, David W. Purcell, Julia Downing, Frank Kaharuza, Jonathan Mermin, Samuel Malamba, and Rebecca Bunnell. 2006. Disclosure of HIV Status and Adherence to Daily Drug Regimens Among HIV-infected Children in Uganda. *AIDS and Behavior* 10 (1): 85–93.

Bledsoe, Caroline, and Uche Isiugo-Abanihe. 1989. "Strategies of Child-Fosterage among Mende Grannies in Sierra Leone." In *Reproduction and Social Organization in Sub-Saharan Africa,* edited by R. J. Lesthaeghe, 442–74. Berkeley: University of California Press.

Bluebond-Langner, Myra. 1978. *The Private Worlds of Dying Children.* Princeton, NJ: Princeton University Press.

Borneman, John. 2001. "Caring and Being Cared For: Displacing Marriage, Kinship, Gender and Sexuality." In *The Ethics of Kinship: Ethnographic Enquiries,* edited by J. Faubion, 29–46. New Jersey: Rowland and Littlefield.

Bornstein, Erica. 2003. *The Spirit of Development: Protestant NGOs, Morality, and Economics in Zimbabwe.* London: Routledge.

———. 2012. *Disquieting Gifts: Humanitarianism in New Delhi.* Stanford, CA: Stanford University Press.

Bornstein, Erica, and Peter Redfield, eds. 2010. *Forces of Compassion: Humanitarianism between Ethics and Politics*. Santa Fe, NM: School for Advanced Research Press.

Bourdieu, Pierre. 1977. *Outline of a Theory of Practice*. Cambridge: Cambridge University Press.

Bowie, Fiona, ed. 2004. *Cross-Cultural Approaches to Adoption*. New York: Routledge.

Boyden, Jo. 1997. "Childhood and the Policy Makers: A Comparative Perspective on the Globalization of Childhood." In *Constructing and Reconstructing Childhood*, edited by A. James and A. Prout, 190–229. Washington, DC: Falmer.

———. 2015. "Epistemological and Ideological Clashes in Research and Policy around Children and Childhood." Paper presented at Third International Conference of the International Childhood and Youth Research Network, European University, Nicosia, Cyprus, June 10.

Brennan, Samantha. 2002. "Children's Choices or Children's Interests: Which Do Their Rights Protect?" In *The Moral and Political Status of Children*, edited by D. Archard and C. M. MacLeod, 53–69. New York: Oxford University Press.

Briggs, Laura. 2012. *Somebody's Children: The Politics of Transracial and Transnational Adoption*. Durham, NC: Duke University Press.

Bunkers, Kelley McCreery, Karen Smith Rotabi, and Benyam Dawit Mezmur. 2012. "Ethiopia at a Critical Juncture in Intercountry Adoption and Traditional Care Practices." In *Intercountry Adoption: Policies, Practices, and Outcomes*, edited by Judith Gibbons and Karen Smith Rotabi, 133–42. Surrey, UK: Ashgate.

Butt, Leslie. 2002. "The Suffering Stranger: Medical Anthropology and International Morality." *Medical Anthropology* 24 (1): 1–24.

Campbell, Alan. 2008. "For Their Own Good: Recruiting Children for Research." *Childhood* 15 (1): 30–49.

Carsten, Janet, ed. 2000. *Cultures of Relatedness: New Approaches to the Study of Kinship*. Cambridge: Cambridge University Press.

———. 2004. *After Kinship: New Departures in Anthropology*. New York: Cambridge University Press.

———. 2011. "Substance and Relationality: Blood in Contexts." *Annual Review of Anthropology* 40 (1): 19–35.

———. 2013. "'Searching for the Truth': Tracing the Moral Properties of Blood in Malaysian Clinical Pathology Labs." *Journal of the Royal Anthropological Institute* 19 (S1):S130–S148. doi: 10.1111/1467-9655.12020.

Cartwright, Lisa. 2005. "'Images of "Waiting Children': Spectatorship and Pity in the Representation of the Global Social Orphan in the 1990s." In *Cultures of Transnational Adoption*, edited by Toby Alice Volkman, 185–214. Durham, NC: Duke University Press.

Cheney, Kristen E. 2007a. "Global Rights Discourse, National Developments, and Local Childhoods: Dilemmas of Childhood and Nationhood in Uganda, East Africa." In *Histoires d'enfant, histoires d'enfance (Stories for Children, Histories of Childhood)*, edited by R. Findlay and S. Salbayre, 47–70. Tours, France: Presses Universitaires François Rabelais.

———. 2007b. *Pillars of the Nation: Child Citizens and Ugandan National Development*. Chicago: University of Chicago Press.

———. 2010. "Expanding Vulnerability, Dwindling Resources: Implications for Orphaned Futures in Uganda." *Childhood in Africa* 2 (1) :8–15.

———. 2012. "Locating Neocolonialism, '"Tradition,' and Human Rights in Uganda's 'Gay Death Penalty.'" *African Studies Review* 55 (2): 77–95.

———. 2014a. "Conflicting Protectionist and Empowerment Models of Children's Rights: Their

Consequences for Uganda's Orphans and Vulnerable Children." In *Children's Lives in an Era of Children's Rights: The Progress of the Convention on the Rights of the Child in Africa*, edited by Afua Twum-Danso and Nicola Ansell, 17–33. New York: Routledge.

———. 2014b. "Giving Children a 'Better Life'? Reconsidering Social Reproduction and Humanitarianism in Intercountry Adoption." *European Journal of Development Research* 26 (2): 247–63.

———. 2015. "Blood Binds: Confronting the Moral and Political Economies of Orphanhood and Adoption in Uganda." *Childhood* 23 (2): 192-206. doi: 10.1177/0907568215602319.

Cheney, Kristen E., and Karen Smith Rotabi. 2014. "'Addicted to Orphans': How the Global Orphan Industrial Complex Jeopardizes Local Child Protection Systems." In *Conflict, Violence and Peace*, vol. 11, *Geographies of Children and Young People*, edited by Christopher Harker, Kathrin Hörschelmann, and Tracey Skelton, 1–19. Singapore: Springer Science + Business Media.

Child Rights Coalition Asia. 2012. "New Optional Protocol to the CRC Officially Signed by States." Accessed February 22. http://www.childrightscoalitionasia.org/new-optional -protocol-to-the-crc-officially-signed-by-states/ [link no longer active].

Child Rights Connect. 2014. "OP3 CRC Is Now In Force." News release. April 21. http://www .childrightsconnect.org/press-release-op3-crc/.

Child Rights International Network (CRIN). 2011. "UN Adopts Complaints Mechanism for Children." December 19. http://www.crin.org/resources/infodetail.asp?ID=26980.

Childs i Foundation. 2013. "Ugandans Adopt NTV Talk Show Part 3." May 31. Accessed April 27, 2016. https://www.youtube.com/watch?v=3_dqXH7o_ng.

Chirwa, Wiseman. 2002. "Social Exclusion and Inclusion: Challenges to Orphan Care in Malawi." *Nordic Journal of African Studies* 11 (1): 93–113.

Chouliaraki, Lilie. 2013. *The Ironic Spectator: Solidarity in the Age of Post-Humanitarianism*. Malden, MA: Polity Press.

Christensen, Pia, and Allison James. 2000. *Research with Children: Perspectives and Practices*. New York: Falmer Press.

Christensen, Pia, and Alan Prout. 2002. "Working with Ethical Symmetry in Social Research with Children." *Childhood* 9 (4): 477–97.

Clifford, James, and George E. Marcus. 1986. *Writing Culture*. Berkeley: University of California Press.

Cole, Jennifer, and Deborah Durham. 2008. "Introduction: Globalization and the Temporality of Children and Youth." In *Figuring the Future: Globalization and Temporalities of Children and Youth*, edited by J. Cole and D. Durham, 3–23. Santa Fe, NM: School for Advanced Research Press.

Cooper, Elizabeth. 2010. "Inheritance and the Intergenerational Transmission of Poverty in Sub-Saharan Africa: Policy Considerations." In *Chronic Poverty Research Centre Working Papers*. Oxford: Chronic Poverty Research Centre.

Culp-Ressler, Tara. 2015. "'Historic' Ruling States That Abstinence-Only Sex Ed Isn't Sex Ed." ThinkProgress. May 13. http://thinkprogress.org/health/2015/05/13/3658139/california -judge-abstinence-only/.

Dahl, Bianca. 2012. "Beyond the Blame Paradigm: Rethinking Witchcraft Gossip and Stigma around HIV-Positive Children in Southeastern Botswana." *African Historical Review* 44 (1): 53–79. doi: 10.1080/17532523.2012.714160.

Davel, Trynie. 2008. "Intercountry Adoption from an African Perspective. In *Children's Rights in Africa: A Legal Perspective*, edited by J. Sloth-Nielsen, 257–77. Hampshire, Eng.: Ashgate.

Davies, Miranda. 2011. "Intercountry Adoption, Children's Rights and the Politics of Rescue." *Adoption and Fostering* 35 (4):50–62. doi: 10.1177/030857591103500406.

de Klerk, Josien. 2012. "The Compassion of Concealment: Silence between Older Caregivers and Dying Patients in the AIDS Era, Northwest Tanzania." *Culture, Health and Sexuality* 14:S27–S38. doi: 10.2307/23524536.

de Waal, Alex, and Nicolas Argenti, eds. 2002. *Young Africa: Realising the Rights of Children and Youth.* Trenton, NJ: Africa World Press.

di Mauro, Diane, and Carole Joffe. 2008. "The Religious Right and the Reshaping of Sexual Policy: Reproductive Rights and Sexuality Education during the Bush Years." In *Moral Panics, Sex Panics: Fear and Fight over Sexual Rights,* edited by G. Herdt. New York: New York University Press.

Dozier, Mary, Charles H. Zeanah, Allison R. Wallin, and Carole Shauffer. 2012. "Institutional Care for Young Children: Review of Literature and Policy Implications." *Social Issues and Policy Review* 6 (1): 1–25. doi: 10.1111/j.1751-2409.2011.01033.x.

Drah, Bright. 2012. "Orphans in Sub-Saharan Africa: The Crisis, the Interventions, and the Anthropologist." *Africa Today* 59 (2): 2–21.

Dubinsky, Karen. 2010. *Babies without Borders: Adoption and Migration across the Americas.* New York: New York University Press.

Ehlers, Louise, and Cheryl Frank. 2008. "Child Participation in Africa." In Sloth-Nielsen, *Children's Rights in Africa,* 111–27.

Englund, Harri. 2006. *Prisoners of Freedom: Human Rights and the African Poor.* Berkeley: University of California Press.

Ennew, Judith. 2002. "Future Generations and Global Standards: Children's Rights at the Start of the Millennium." In *Exotic No More: Anthropology on the Front Lines,* edited by J. MacClancy, 338–50. Chicago: University of Chicago Press.

Epstein, Helen. 2007. *The Invisible Cure: Why We Are Losing the Fight against AIDS in Africa.* New York: Picador.

Evans, Rosalind. 2007. "The Impact of Concepts of Childhood on Children's Participation in Bhutanese Refugee Camps." *Children, Youth and Environments* 17 (1): 148–74.

Executive Board of the American Anthropological Association. 1947. "Statement on Human Rights." *American Anthropologist* 49 (4): 539–543. doi: 10.1525/aa.1947.49.4.02a00020.

Falk Moore, Sally. 1994. *Anthropology and Africa: Changing Perspectives on a Changing Scene.* Charlottesville: University of Virginia Press.

Farmer, Paul. (1992) 2006. *AIDS and Accusation: Haiti and the Geography of Blame.* Berkeley: University of California Press.

Fass, Paula S. 2008. "Childhood and Youth as an American/Global Experience in the Context of the Past." In Cole and Durham, *Figuring the Future,* 25–47.

Fassin, Didier. 2005. "Compassion and Repression: The Moral Economy of Immigration Policies in France." *Cultural Anthropology* 20 (3): 362–387.

———. 2007a. "Humanitarianism as a Politics of Life." *Public Culture* 19 (3): 499–520.

———. 2007b. *When Bodies Remember: Experiences and Politics of AIDS in South Africa.* Berkeley: University of California Press.

———. 2013. "Children as Victims: The Moral Economy of Childhood in the Times of AIDS." In *When People Come First: Critical Studies in Global Health,* edited by J. Biehl and A. Petryna, 109–32. Princeton, NJ: Princeton University Press.

Feldman, Ilana, and Miriam Ticktin, eds. 2010. *In the Name of Humanity: The Government of Threat and Care.* Durham, NC: Duke University Press.

Ferguson, Anne, and Andrea Freidus. 2007. "Orphan Care in Malawi: Examining the Trans-national Images and Discourses of Humanitarianism." Paper presented at American Anthropological Association Meetings. Washington, DC.

Ferguson, James. 1994. *The Anti-Politics Machine: "Development," Depoliticization, and Bureaucratic Power in Lesotho*. Minneapolis: University of Minnesota Press.

———. 2006. *Global Shadows: Africa in the Neoliberal World Order*. Durham, NC: Duke University Press.

Fisher, William F. 1997. "Doing Good? The Politics and Antipolitics of NGO Practices." *Annual Review of Anthropology* 26:439–64.

Foster, Geoff, Carol Levine, and John Williamson, eds. 2005. *A Generation at Risk: The Global Impact of HIV/AIDS on Orphans and Vulnerable Children*. New York: Cambridge University Press.

Frankel, Sam. 2007. "Researching Children's Morality: Developing Research Methods That Allow Children's Involvement in Discourses Relevant to Their Everyday Lives." *Childhoods Today* 1 (1): 1–25.

Franklin, Bob, ed. 1986. *The Rights of Children*. Oxford: Basil Blackwell.

Freidus, Andrea, and Anne Ferguson. 2013. "Malawi's Orphans: The Role of Transnational Humanitarian Organizations." In *Vulnerable Children: Global Challenges in Education, Health, Well-Being, and Child Rights*, edited by Deborah Jean Johnson, DeBrenna LaFa Agbényiga, and Robert K. Hitchcock, 203–15. New York: Springer.

Fussell, Elizabeth, and Margaret E. Greene. 2002. "Demographic Trends Affecting Youth around the World." In *The World's Youth: Adolescence in Eight Regions of the Globe*, edited by B. B. Brown, R. W. Larson, and T. S. Saraswathi, 21–60. New York: Cambridge University Press.

Geertz, Clifford. 1998. "Deep Hanging Out." *New York Review of Books*. October 22. http://www.nybooks.com/articles/1998/10/22/deep-hanging-out/.

Geiselhart, Klaus, Thando D. Gwebu, and Fred Kruger. 2008. "Children, Adolescents and the HIV and AIDS Pandemic: Changing Inter-Generational Relationships and Intra-Family Communication Patterns in Botswana." *Children, Youth and Environments* 18 (1): 99–125.

Geschiere, Peter. 2003. "Witchcraft as the Dark Side of Kinship: Dilemmas of Social Security in New Contexts." *Etnofoor* 16 (1): 43–61.

Global Initiative to End All Corporal Punishment of Children. 2016. *Corporal Punishment of Children in Uganda*. Accessed May 2. http://www.endcorporalpunishment.org/assets/pdfs/states-reports/Uganda.pdf.

Goody, Esther. 1982. *Parenthood and Social Reproduction: Fostering and Occupational Roles in West Africa*. New York: Cambridge University Press.

Goody, Jack, and Esther Goody. 1969. "The Circulation of Women and Children in Northern Ghana." In *Comparative Studies in Kinship*, edited by J. Goody, 184–215. Palo Alto, CA: Stanford University Press.

Government of Uganda. 1997. *The Children Act*. Kampala: Government of Uganda.

Groundwater-Smith, Susan, Sue Dockett, and Dorothy Bottrell. 2015. *Participatory Research with Children and Young People*. London: Sage.

Gruskin, Sofia, and Daniel Tarantola. 2005. "Human Rights and Children Affected by HIV/AIDS." In Foster, Levine, and Williamson, *A Generation at Risk*, 134–58.

Guest, Emma. 2003. *Children of AIDS: Africa's Orphan Crisis*. 2d ed. London: Pluto Press.

Hansen, Karen T. 2008. "Localities and Sites of Youth Agency in Lusaka." In *Youth and the City in the Global South*, ed. K. T. Hansen, 98–124. Bloomington: Indiana University Press.

Hanson, Karl, and Olga Nieuwenhuys, eds. 2013. *Reconceptualizing Children's Rights in International Development: Living Rights, Social Justice, Translations.* Cambridge: Cambridge University Press.

Hardon, Anita, and Deborah Posel. 2012. "Secrecy as Embodied Practice: Beyond the Confessional Imperative." *Culture, Health and Sexuality* 14 (sup1): S1–S13. doi: 10.1080/13691058.2012.726376.

Henderson, Patricia C. 2006. "South African AIDS Orphans: Examining Assumptions around Vulnerability from the Perspective of Rural Children and Youth." *Childhood* 13 (3): 303–27.

Hirschfeld, Lawrence. 2002. "Why Don't Anthropologists Like Children?" *American Anthropologist* 104 (2): 611–27.

Hoffman, Diane M. 2012. "Saving Children, Saving Haiti? Child Vulnerability and Narratives of the Nation." *Childhood* 19 (2):155–68. doi: 10.1177/0907568211415297.

Honwana, A., and de Boeck, F., eds. 2005. *Makers and Breakers: Children and Youth in Postcolonial Africa.* Trenton, NJ: Africa World Press.

Howell, Signe. 2006. *The Kinning of Foreigners: Transnational Adoption in a Global Perspective.* New York: Berghahn Books.

———. 2009. "Adoption of the Unrelated Child: Some Challenges to the Anthropological Study of Kinship." *Annual Review of Anthropology* 38 (1):149–66. doi: doi:10.1146/annurev.anthro.37.081407.085115.

Huijsmans, Roy, and Simon Baker. 2012. "Child Trafficking: 'Worst Form' of Child Labour, or Worst Approach to Young Migrants?" *Development and Change* 43 (4): 919–46.

Human Rights Watch/Africa. 2005. *The Less They Know, the Better: Abstinence-Only HIV/AIDS Programs in Uganda.* New York: Human Rights Watch.

Hunter, Mark. 2010. *Love in the Time of AIDS: Inequality, Gender, and Rights in South Africa.* Bloomington: Indiana University Press.

Hunter, S. S. 1990. "Orphans as a Window on the AIDS Epidemic in Sub-Saharan Africa: Initial Results and Implications of a Study in Uganda." *Social Science and Medicine* 31 (6): 681–90.

International Labour Office (ILO). 2012. *The Youth Employment Crisis: Time for Action; Report Submitted to the Delegates of the 101st International Labour Labour Conference for General Discussion.* Vol. 5. Geneva: International Labour Office.

Invernizzi, Antonella, and Brian Milne. 2002. "Are Children Entitled to Contribute to International Policy Making? A Critical View of Children's Participation in the International Campaign for the Elimination of Child Labour." *International Journal of Children's Rights* 10 (4): 403–31.

———. 2005. "Introduction: Children's Citizenship; A New Discourse?" *Journal of Social Sciences* (9): 1–6.

James, Allison. 2007. "Giving Voice to Children's Voices: Practices and Problems, Pitfalls and Potentials." *American Anthropologist* 109 (2): 261–72.

———. 2011. "To Be (Come) or Not to Be (Come): Understanding Children's Citizenship." *The Annals of the American Academy of Political and Social Science* 633 (1): 167–79.

James, Allison, Chris Jenks, and Alan Prout, eds. 1998. *Theorizing Childhood.* Oxford: Polity Press.

Jenks, Chris. 1996. *Childhood.* New York: Routledge.

Joint Learning Initiative on Children and HIV/AIDS. 2009. *Home Truths: Facing the Facts on Children, AIDS, and Poverty.* Geneva: Association François-Xavier Bagnoud—FXB International.

Joyce, Kathryn. 2013a. *The Child Catchers: Rescue, Trafficking, and the New Gospel of Adoption.* New York: Public Affairs.

———. 2013b. "Hana's Story: An Adoptee's Tragic Fate, and How It Could Happen Again." *Slate,* November 9. http://www.slate.com/articles/double_x/doublex/2013/11/hana_williams_the _tragic_death_of_an_ethiopian_adoptee_and_how_it_could.html.

Kabadaki, Kyama K. 2001. "The Feminization of Poverty in Rural Sub-Saharan Africa." In *Social Problems in Africa: New Visions,* edited by A. Rwomire, 93–110. Westport, CT: Praeger.

Kamusiime, Annah, and Auma Okwany. Forthcoming. "Foregrounding the Tensions and Silences in Policies for Student-Mothers in Uganda and Kenya." *Childhood in Africa.*

Kaoma, Kapya John. 2012. *Colonizing African Values—How the U.S. Christian Right is Transforming Sexual Politics in Africa: Executive Summary.* Somerville, MA: Political Research Associates.

Karimi, Faith, Samson Ntale, and Greg Botelho. 2016. "Uganda Leader Museveni Declared Winner—Despite Issues, Tensions." CNN. February 21. http://www.cnn.com/2016/02/20/africa/ uganda-election/.

Kasozi, Ephraim. 2016. "Former AG Nyombi Pokes Holes in New Children Act." *Daily Monitor.* March 22. http://www.monitor.co.ug/News/National/Former-AG-Nyombi-pokes-holes-in -new-Children-Act/-/688334/3127456/-/gcu69o/-/index.html.

Katabira, Elly T., Moses R. Kamya, Israel Kalyesubula, and Alice Namale. 2008. *National Antiretroviral Treatment and Care Guidelines for Adults, Adolescents, and Children.* Kampala, Uganda: Ministry of Health.

Katz, Cindi. 2003. "The State Goes Home: Children, Social Reproduction, and the Terrors of 'Hypervigilance.'" Paper presented at American Anthropological Association Annual Meeting, Chicago, November 20.

Kaufmann, Jeffrey, and Annie Phillippe Rabodoarimiadana. 2003. "Making Kin of Historians and Anthropologists: Fictive Kinship in Fieldwork Methodology." *History in Africa* 30:179–94.

Kelly, Michael J. 2003. "Reducing the Vulnerability of Africa's Children to HIV/AIDS." In *The Children of Africa Confront AIDS: From Vulnerability to Possibility,* edited by Arvind Singhal and W. Stephen Howard, 59–84. Athens: Ohio University Press.

Kendall, Nancy. 2013. *The Sex Education Debates.* Chicago: University of Chicago Press.

Kendrick, Maureen, and Doris Kakuru. 2012. "Funds of Knowledge in Child-Headed Households: A Ugandan Case Study." *Childhood* 19 (3): 397–413.

Kilbride, Philip L., and Janet C. Kilbride. 1990. *Changing Family Life in East Africa: Women and Children at Risk.* University Park: Pennsylvania State University Press.

Kleinman, Arthur, Veena Das, and Margaret Lock, eds. 1997. *Social Suffering.* Berkeley: University of California Press.

Lemma, Tarikuwa. 2014. "International Adoption Made Me a Commodity, Not a Daughter." October 31. *Guardian.* http://www.theguardian.com/commentisfree/2014/oct/31/international -adoption-made-me-a-commodity-not-a-daughter.

Liebel, Manfred. 2012. *Children's Rights from Below: Cross-Cultural Perspectives.* New York: Palgrave-MacMillan.

Lowenthal, Elizabeth D., Haruna B. Jibril, Mmapula L. Sechele, Keofentse Mathuba, Ontibile Tshume, and Gabriel M. Anabwani. 2014. "Disclosure of HIV Status to HIV-infected Children in a Large African Treatment Center: Lessons Learned in Botswana." *Children and Youth Services Review* 45:143–49. doi: http://dx.doi.org/10.1016/j.childyouth.2014.03.031.

Madhavan, Sangeetha. 2004. "Fosterage Patterns in the Age of AIDS: Continuity and Change." *Social Science and Medicine* 58 (7): 1443–54.

Mahon, Margaret A. 2011. "Death in the Lives of Children." In *Children's Understanding of Death*, edited by V. Talwar, P. L. Harris, and M. Schleifer, 61–97. New York: Cambridge University Press.

Mahon, Rianne. 2010. "After Neo-Liberalism? The OECD, the World Bank and the Child." *Global Social Policy* 10 (2): 172–92.

Mains, Daniel. 2013. *Hope Is Cut: Youth, Unemployment, and the Future in Urban Ethiopia*. Philadelphia: Temple University Press.

Malinga, Joseph. 2010. "Defilement Crime on the Rise in Uganda." *Guardian*, October 7. http://www.guardian.co.uk/katine/2010/oct/06/uganda-katine-defilement.

Malkki, Liisa. 2010. "Children, Humanity, and the Infantilization of Peace." In Feldman and Ticktin, *In the Name of Humanity*, 58–85.

Mannheim, Karl. 1982. "The Problem of Generations." In *The Sociology of Childhood: Essential Readings*, edited by Chris Jenks, 256–69. London: Batsford Academic and Educational Limited.

Marre, Diana, and Laura Briggs, eds. 2009. *International Adoption: Global Inequalities and the Circulation of Children*. New York: New York University Press.

Mayall, Berry. 1999. "Children and Childhood." In *Critical Issues in Social Research: Power and Prejudice*, edited by S. Hood, B. Mayall, and S. Oliver, 10–24. Philadelphia: Open University Press.

McEwen, C, and D. Bek. 2006. "(Re)politicizing Empowerment: Lessons from the South African Wine Industry." *Geoforum* 37:1021–34.

McNeil, Donald G. Jr. 2015. "U.S. Push for Abstinence in Africa Is Seen as Failure Against H.I.V." *New York Times*, February 26. http://www.nytimes.com/2015/02/27/health/american-hiv -battle-in-africa-said-to-falter.html.

Meintjes, Helen, and Sonja Giese. 2006. "Spinning the Epidemic: The Making of Mythologies of Orphanhood in the Context of AIDS." *Childhood* 13 (3): 407–30.

Michael, Sarah. 2004. *Undermining Development: The Absence of Power among Local NGOs in Africa, African Issues*. Bloomington: Indiana University Press.

Milne, Brian. 2005. "Is 'Participation' as It Is Described by the United Nations Convention on the Rights of the Child (UNCRC) the Key to Children's Citizenship?" *Journal of Social Sciences* (special issue no. 9): 31–42.

Moyer, Eileen. 2012. "Faidha gani? What's the point: HIV and the Logics of (Non-)Disclosure among Young Activists in Zanzibar." *Culture, Health and Sexuality* 14 (sup1): S67–S79. doi: 10.1080/13691058.2012.662524.

Murdoch, Lydia. 2006. *Imagined Orphans: Poor Families, Child Welfare, and Contested Citizenship in London*. New Brunswick: Rutgers University Press.

Mutua, Kagendo, and Beth Blue Swadener, eds. 2004. *Decolonizing Research in Cross-Cultural Contexts: Critical Personal Narratives*. Albany: State University of New York Press.

Naker, Dipak. 2007. "From Rhetoric to Practice: Bridging the Gap Between What We Believe and What We Do." *Children, Youth, and Environments* 17 (3): 146–58.

Namubiru Mukasa, Sylvia. 2013. "Applying the Principle of the Best Interests of the Child in Inter-Country Legal Guardianship and Adoption Matters: Experiences of the Family Court in Uganda." Human Rights, Gender and Conflict: Social Justice Perspectives Master of Arts thesis, International Institute of Social Studies, Erasmus University.

Nelson, Kim Park. 2010. "The Horror of Adoption: The Mother, the Other and the Other Mother in *The Ring/The Ring 2, Silent Hill, The Abandoned* and *The Orphan.*" Paper presented at conference Adoption: Secret Histories, Public Policies, Massachusetts Institute of Technology, Cambridge, MA, April 29–May 2.

Notermans, Catrien. 2004. "Fosterage and the Politics of Marriage and Kinship in East Cameroon." In *Cross-Cultural Approaches to Adoption*, edited by F. Bowie, 48–63. New York: Routledge.

———. 2008. "The Emotional World of Kinship: Children's Experiences of Fosterage in East Cameroon." *Childhood* 15 (3): 355–77.

Ntarangwi, Mwenda, David Mills, and Mustafa Babiker, eds. 2006. *African Anthropologies: History, Critique, and Practice.* New York: Zed Books in association with CODESRIA.

NTV Uganda. 2013. "Taken and Never Returned: When Adoption Profits the Middleman." April 19. https://www.youtube.com/watch?v=yEeDL70WKOA&list=PLPz47e2di8dP7rcr KxbsqoQqQk2wZ1lrk&index=4.

Nyambedha, Erick Otieno, and Jens Aagaard-Hansen. 2003. "Changing Place, Changing Position: Orphans' Movements in a Community with High HIV/AIDS Prevalence in Western Kenya." In *Children's Places: Cross-Cultural Perspectives*, edited by Karen Fog Olwig and Eva Gullov, 162–76. New York: Routledge.

Nyombi, Peter. 2016. "Public Notice on Legal Adoption/Guardianship Allegations." *New Vision.* February 26. http://www.newvision.co.ug/digital_assets/68366136-de07-48cc-9fe8-f656292 08701/ST1NV290216.p02-legal-31.pdf.

Oburu, Paul Odhiambo. 2004. *Social Adjustment of Kenyan Orphaned Grandchildren, Perceived Caregiving Stress and Discipline Strategies Used by their Fostering Grandmothers.* Goteborg, Sweden: Department of Psychology.

Oleke, Christopher, Astrid Blystad, Karen Marie Moland, Ole Bjorn Rekdal, and Kristian Heggenhougen. 2006. "The Varying Vulnerability of African Orphans: The Case of the Langi, Northern Uganda." *Childhood* 13 (2): 267–84.

Oleke, Christopher, Astrid Blystad, and Ole Bjorn Rekdal. 2005. "'When the Obvious Brother Is Not There': Political and Cultural Contexts of the Orphan Challenge in Northern Uganda." *Social Science and Medicine* 61 (12): 2628–38.

Parsons, Ross. 2005. "Grief-Stricken: Zimbabwean Children in Everyday Extremity and the Ethics of Research." *Anthropology Southern Africa* 28 (3–4): 73–77.

———. 2012. *Growing Up with HIV in Zimbabwe: One Day This Will All Be Over.* Woodbridge: James Currey.

Patterson, Amy S. 2003. "AIDS, Orphans, and the Future of Democracy in Africa." In Singhal and Howard, *Children of Africa Confront AIDS*, 13–39.

Pease, Bob. 2002. "Rethinking Empowerment: A Postmodern Reappraisal for Emancipatory Practice." *British Journal of Social Work* 32 (2): 135–47.

Phiri, Stanley Ngalazu, and David Tolfree. 2005. "Family and Community-Based Care for Children Affected by HIV/AIDS: Strengthening the Front Line Response." In Foster, Levine, and Williamson, *A Generation at Risk*, 11–36.

POLICY Project. 2005. *Executive Summary: OVC RAAAP Initiative Final Report.* Washington, DC: US Agency for International Development (USAID).

Powell, Mary Ann, and Anne B. Smith. 2009. "Children's Participation Rights in Research." *Childhood* 16 (1): 124–42.

President's Emergency Plan for AIDS Relief. 2012. *PEPFAR Blueprint: Creating an AIDS-Free Generation.* Washington, DC: Office of the Global AIDS Coordinator.

Pryor, John, and Joseph Ghartey Ampiah. 2004. "Listening to Voices in the Village: Collaborating through Data Chains." In Mutua and Swadener, *Decolonizing Research in Cross-Cultural Contexts*, 159–78.

Pupavac, Vanessa. 2001. "Misanthropy without Borders: The International Children's Rights Regime." *Disasters* 25 (2): 95–112. doi: 10.1111/1467–7717.00164.

Quiroz, Pamela Anne. 2012. "Cultural Tourism in Transnational Adoption: 'Staged Authenticity' and Its Implications for Adopted Children." *Journal of Family Issues* 33 (4): 527–55. doi: 10.1177/0192513X11418179.

Ranger, Terence O., ed. 2008. *Evangelical Christianity and Democracy in Africa*. Oxford: Oxford University Press.

Richter, Linda M., and Amy Norman. 2010. "AIDS Orphan Tourism: A Threat to Young Children in Residential Care." *Vulnerable Children and Youth Studies* 5 (3): 217–29. doi: 10.1080/17450128.2010.487124.

Riley, Mark. 2012. *Baseline Study: The State of Institutional Care in Uganda*. Kampala: Uganda Ministry of Gender, Labour and Social Development.

———. 2014. "Training Changing Lives of Children in Uganda." Uniting for Children. June 19. http://unitingforchildren.org/2014/06/changing-lives-in-uganda/.

Robson, Elsbeth, and Nicola Ansell. 2000. "Young Carers in Southern Africa: Exploring Stories from Zimbabwean Secondary School Students." In *Children's Geographies*, edited by S. Holloway and G. Valentine, 174–93. New York: Routledge.

Roby, Jini L. 2011. *Children in Informal Alternative Care*. New York: UNICEF Child Protection Section. June. http://www.unicef.org/protection/Informal_care_discussion_paper_final.pdf.

Roby, Jini L., and Stacey A. Shaw. 2006. "The African Orphan Crisis and International Adoption." *Social Work* 51 (3): 199–210.

Rogers, Annie G., Mary E. Casey, Jennifer Ekert, James Holland, Victoria Nakkula, and Nuril Sheinberg. 1999. "An Interpretive Poetics of Languages of the Unsayable." In *Making Meaning of Narratives*, edited by R. Josselson and A. Lieblich, 77–106. London: Sage.

Rose, Laurel R. 2005. "Orphans' Land Rights in Post-War Rwanda: The Problem of Guardianship." *Development and Change* 36 (5): 911–36.

Ross, Fiona C. 2001. "Speech and Silence: Women's Testimony in the First Five Weeks of Public Hearings of the South African Truth and Reconciliation Commission." In *Remaking a World: Violence, Social Suffering, and Recovery*, edited by Veena Das, Pamela Reynolds, and Mamphela Ramphele, 250–80. Berkeley: University of California Press.

Save the Children. 2006. *Child Rights Programming: How to Apply Rights-Based Approaches to Programming—A Handbook for Internationals*. London: Save the Children Alliance Members.

Schatz, Enid J. 2007. "'Taking Care of My Own Blood': Older Women's Relationships to Their Households in Rural South Africa." *Scandinavian Journal of Public Health* 69:147–54.

Scherz, China. 2014. *Having People, Having Heart: Charity, Sustainable Development, and Problems of Dependence in Central Uganda*. Chicago: University of Chicago Press.

Schumaker, Lyn. 2001. *Africanizing Anthropology: Fieldwork, Networks, and the Making of Cultural Knowledge in Central Africa*. Durham, NC: Duke University Press.

Schwartzman, Helen B., ed. 2001. *Children and Anthropology: Perspectives for the 21st Century*. Westport, CT: Bergin and Garvey.

Schwarzschild, Todd. 2013. "Red Flags Wave over Uganda's Adoption Boom." CNN. March 2. http://edition.cnn.com/2013/02/27/world/africa/wus-uganda-adoptions.

Seeley, Janet. 2014. *HIV and East Africa: Thirty Years in the Shadow of an Epidemic*. New York: Routledge.

Selman, Peter. 2013a. *Key Tables for Intercountry Adoption: Receiving States and States of Origin 2003–2012*. Newcastle: Newcastle University.

———. 2013b. "One Million Children Moving: The Demography of Intercountry Adoption." Paper presented at Fourth International Conference on Adoption Research (ICAR4), Bilbao, Spain, July 7–11.

Sherr, Lorraine, Rebecca Varrall, Joanne Mueller, Linda Richter, Angela Wakhweya, Michele Adato, Mark Belsey, Upjeet Chandan, Scott Drimie, Mary Haour-Knipe Victoria Hosegood, Jose Kimou, Sangeetha Madhavan, Vuyiswa Mathambo, and Chris Desmond. 2008. "A Systematic Review on the Meaning of the Concept 'AIDS Orphan': Confusion over Definitions and Implications for Care." *AIDS Care* 20 (5): 527–36.

Sikstrom, Laura. 2014. ""Without the Grandparents, Life Is Difficult': Social Hierarchy and Therapeutic Trajectories for Children Living with HIV in Rural Northern Malawi." *Children and Youth Services Review* 45:47–54. doi: http://dx.doi.org/10.1016/j.childyouth.2014.03.037.

Simmel, Georg. 1906. "The Sociology of Secrecy and of Secret Societies." *American Journal of Sociology* 11 (4): 441–98. doi: 10.2307/2762562.

Sloth-Nielsen, Julia, and Benyam D. Mezmur. 2008. "HIV/Aids and Children's Rights in Law and Policy in Africa: Confronting Hydra Head On." In Sloth-Nielsen, *Children's Rights in Africa*, 279–98.

Smolin, David. 2010. "Child Laundering and the Hague Convention on Intercountry Adoption: The Future and Past of Intercountry Adoption." *University of Louisville Law Review* 48 (3): 441–98.

Stephens, Sharon, ed. 1995. *Children and the Politics of Culture*. Princeton, NJ: Princeton University Press.

Stillwaggon, Eileen. 2006. *AIDS and the Ecology of Poverty*. Oxford: Oxford University Press.

Stone, Linda, ed. 2001. *New Directions in Anthropological Kinship*. Oxford: Rowman and Littlefield.

Suski, Laura. 2009. "Children, Suffering and the Humanitarian Appeal." In *Humanitarianism and Suffering: The Mobilization of Empathy*, edited by Richard A. Wilson and Richard D. Brown, 202–22. New York: Cambridge University Press.

Susser, Ida. 2009. *AIDS, Sex, and Culture: Global Politics and Survival in Southern Africa*. West Sussex, UK: Wiley-Blackwell.

Swift, Anthony, and Stan Maher. 2008. *Growing Pains: How Poverty and AIDS are Undermining Childhood*. London: Panos.

Tamasane, Tsiliso, and Judith Head. 2010. "The Quality of Material Care Provided by Grandparents for their Orphaned Grandchildren in the Context of HIV/AIDS and Poverty: A Study of Kopanong Municipality, Free State." *Journal of Social Aspects of HIV/AIDS (SAHARA)* 7 (2): 76–84.

Taylor, Nicola J., and Anne B. Smith, eds. 2009. *Children as Citizens? International Voices; Childwatch International Citizenship Study Group*. Dunedin, New Zealand: Otago University Press.

Thornton, Robert J. 2008. *Unimagined Community: Sex, Networks, and AIDS in Uganda and South Africa*. Berkeley: University of California Press.

Uganda AIDS Commission. 2014. *HIV and AIDS Uganda Country Progress Report 2013*. Kampala: Uganda AIDS Commission.

Uganda Ministry of Gender, Labour and Social Development. 2004. *National Orphans and Vulnerable Children Policy*. Kampala: Ministry of Gender, Labour and Social Development.

———. 2011. *National Strategic Programme Plan of Interventions for Orphans and Other Vulnerable Children 2011/12–2015/16*. Kampala: Ministry of Gender, Labour and Social Development.

———. 2013. "OVCMiS." Accessed July 2. http://www.mglsd.go.ug/ovcmis/index.php (content no longer available).

Uganda Ministry of Gender, Labour and Social Development; Uganda Child Rights NGO Network; and UNICEF—Uganda Office. 2008. *The National Child Participation Guide for Uganda*, edited by Uganda Ministry of Gender, Labour and Social Development.

Uganda Ministry of Health and ICF International. 2012. *2011 Uganda AIDS Indicator Survey: Key Findings*. Calverton, MD: MOH and ICF International.

UNAIDS. 2010. *Global Report: UNAIDS Report on the Global AIDS Epidemic 2010*. Geneva: Joint United Nations Programme on HIV/AIDS (UNAIDS).

———. 2013. *Getting to Zero: HIV in Eastern and Southern Africa*. Johannesburg, South Africa: Joint United Nations Programme on HIV/AIDS (UNAIDS).

———. 2015. "Leaders from Around the World Are All In to End the AIDS Epidemic among Adolescents." News release. February 17. http://www.unaids.org/en/resources/presscentre/pressreleaseandstatementarchive/2015/february/20150217_PR_all-in.

UNICEF. 2003. *Africa's Orphaned Generations*. New York: United Nations Children's Fund (UNICEF).

———. 2005. *Convention on the Rights of the Child: Protecting and Realizing Children's Rights*. Updated May 19, 2014. http://www.unicef.org/crc/index_protecting.html.

———. 2006. *Africa's Orphaned and Vulnerable Generations: Children Affected by AIDS*. New York: UNICEF, UNAIDS, and PEPFAR.

———. 2010. "UNICEF's Position on Inter-Country Adoption." July 22. http://www.unicef.org/media/media_55412.html.

———. 2011. *End Placing Children under Three Years in Institutions—A Call to Action*. New York: UNICEF.

———. 2012. *Countdown to Zero: Elimination of New HIV Infections among Children by 2015 and Keeping Their Mothers Alive*. New York: UNICEF.

———. 2013. "Statistics." Accessed July 2. http://www.unicef.org/infobycountry/uganda_statistics.html.

———. 2014. *Children, Adolescents and AIDS: 2014 Statistical Update*. New York: UNICEF.

———. n.d.a. *Introduction to the Convention on the Rights of the Child: Definition of Key Terms*. http://www.unicef.org/crc/files/Definitions.pdf.

———. n.d.b. *Fact Sheet: The Right to Participation*. http://www.unicef.org/crc/files/Right-to-Participation.pdf.

UNICEF and UNAIDS. 2016. "Uganda: Adolescent HIV Trends and Distribution of Adolescent AIDS-Related Deaths." Accessed April 22. http://allintoendadolescentaids.org/wp-content/uploads/2015/02/Uganda.pdf.

United Nations. 1989. "United Nations Convention on the Rights of the Child." United Nations General Assembly, November 20, 1989.

———. 2000. "United Nations Millennium Declaration." September 8. http://www.un.org/millennium/declaration/ares552e.htm.

United Nations Human Rights Office of the High Commissioner. 2016. "Optional Protocol to the Convention on Rights of the Child on a Communication Procedure." May 2. http://www.ohchr.org/Documents/HRBodies/CRC/OHCHR_Map_CRC-OP-IC.pdf.

US Congress. 2013. Children in Families First Act of 2013. S.R. 1530, 113th Cong.

Urban, Greg. 1996. *Metaphysical Community: The Interplay of the Senses and the Intellect*. Austin: University of Texas Press.

Valentin, Karen, and Lotte Meinert. 2009. "The Adult North and the Young South: Reflections on the Civilizing Mission of Children's Rights." *Anthropology Today* 25 (3): 23–28.

Vernooij, Eva, and Anita Hardon. 2013. "'What Mother Wouldn't Want to Save Her Baby?' HIV Testing and Counselling Practices in a Rural Ugandan Antenatal Clinic." *Culture, Health and Sexuality* 15 (sup 4): S553–S566. doi: 10.1080/13691058.2012.758314.

Voelkl, Hanna T. 2012. "Developing an Understanding of the Experience of Children with International Short-Term Volunteer Tourists—A Case Study of an Orphanage Project in Ghana." MA thesis, School of Health Sciences and Social Care, Brunel University.

Walker, Chris, and Morgan Hartley. 2013. "Cambodia's Orphan-Industrial Complex." *Atlantic*, June 3.

Wandera, Alfred Nyongesa. 2009. "Global Fund Hails Cheeye's Conviction." [Kampala, Uganda], *Daily Monitor*, April 14.

Waugh, S. 2003. "Parental Views on Disclosure of Diagnosis to their HIV-Positive Children." *AIDS Care* 15 (2): 169–76.

Webb, Douglas. 2005. "Interventions to Support Children Affected by HIV/AIDS: Priority Areas for Future Research." In Foster, Levine, and Williamson, *A Generation at Risk*, 232–53.

Weismantel, Mary. 1995. "Making Kin: Kinship Theory and Zumbagua Adoptions." *American Ethnologist* 22 (4): 586–704.

West, Andy. 2007. "Power Relationships and Adult Resistance to Children's Participation." *Children, Youth and Environments* 17 (1): 123–35.

West, Harry G. 2007. *Ethnographic Sorcery*. Chicago: University of Chicago Press.

Whiting, John, and Beatrice Whiting. 1975. *Children of Six Cultures: A Psycho-Cultural Analysis*. Cambridge, MA: Harvard University Press.

Whyte, Susan R., ed. 2014. *Second Chances: Surviving AIDS in Uganda*. Durham, NC: Duke University Press.

Williamson, John, and Aaron Greenberg. 2010. "Families, Not Orphanages." In *Better Care Network Working Paper*. New York: Better Care Network.

Winsor, Morgan. 2016. "Who Will Succeed Uganda's President? Museveni's Controversial Re-Election Could Mean Political, Economic Instability." *International Business Times*. February 24. http://www.ibtimes.com/who-will-succeed-ugandas-president-musevenis-controversial-re-election-could-mean-2320005.

Wood, Bronwyn E. 2013. "Participatory Capital: Bourdieu and Citizenship Education in Diverse School Communities." *British Journal of Sociology of Education* 35 (4): 578–597. doi: 10.1080/01425692.2013.777209.

Woodman, Dan, and Johanna Wyn. 2014. *Youth and Generation: Rethinking Change and Inequality in the Lives of Young People*. London: Sage.

World Bank. 2005. "OVC (Orphans and Other Vulnerable Children)," in OVC Toolkit, 2nd ed. http://info.worldbank.org/etools/docs/library/164047/howknow/definitions.htm.

World Health Organization. 2011. *Guideline on HIV Disclosure Counselling for Children up to 12 Years of Age*. Geneva: World Health Organization.

Yngvesson, Barbara. 2010. *Belonging in an Adopted World: Race, Identity, and Transnational Adoption*. Chicago: University of Chicago Press.

Young, Robert J. C. 2003. *Postcolonialism: A Very Short Introduction*. Oxford: Oxford University Press.

Zelizer, Viviana A. 1985. *Pricing the Priceless Child: The Changing Value of Children*. New York: Basic Books.

Index

Page numbers in boldface refer to figures.

abstinence education, 19–21, 23, 37–38, 116, 184–85; as part of ABC approach, 37, 184. *See also* faith-based organizations; HIV/AIDS; President's Emergency Plan for AIDS Relief (PEPFAR); sexual education

adoption: alternative care models, 159, 162, 163–64, 165, 168, 172, 176, 185–86, 218n10, 218n13; and child trafficking, 10, 95–97, 159, 161–63, 170; domestic (within Uganda), 156–57, 166–77; intercountry (international), 10, 156–59, 161–65, 168, 170–76, 186, 218n9, 219nn17–18, 219n24: from China, 162; from Ethiopia, 161–62, 172; from Russia, 162; from Uganda, 162–65, 172–76. *See also* child trafficking; faith-based organizations; fosterage, of OVC; orphanages; orphans and vulnerable children (OVC)

African Charter on the Rights and Welfare of the Child (ACRWC), 45–46

African Training, Research, and Innovation Network (A-TRAIN), 63–65, **64**, 81. *See also* youth participatory research

AIDS. *See* HIV/AIDS

AIDS-Free Generation, 22–23, 183

All In to End Adolescent AIDS (UNAIDS/UNICEF), 183–84. *See also* HIV/AIDS: and adolescents; UNAIDS; UNICEF

alternative care, 168, 176, 185

Alternative Care for Children in Uganda, 162, 165, 218n10, 218n13. *See also* adoption: alternative care models; orphanages

anthropology: American Anthropological Association, 47; and history of colonialism, 31, 71–73; and participatory research, 58–62, 82–83; and study of children, 31, 35, 47, 58–59, 60–62, 115, 132–33, 155; and study of kinship, 35, 121, 124, 132–33, 138, 152–55, 170; and Universal Declaration of Human Rights, 47. *See also* ethnography, child-centered; youth participatory research

antiretrovirals (ARVs), 8, 13–14, 17–18, 20, 22, 23, 109, 110, 116, 118–20, 128, 195, 197, 203, 205, 215n2 (chap. 1), 217n4 (chap. 6); and post-ARV generation, 7, 8, 9–10, 13–15, **14**, 17 18, 87, 106, 107, 181–84. *See also* HIV/AIDS

antiretroviral treatment (ART). *See* antiretrovirals (ARVs)

Baxter, Jane (archaeologist), 14

Bornstein, Erica, 33

Botswana: and disclosure of HIV status and death to children, 115; success in reducing mother-to-child transmission, 23

Bukenya, Stuart, 163, 173. *See also* adoption: intercountry; child trafficking

Bush, George W., administration, 37. *See also* President's Emergency Plan for AIDS Relief (PEPFAR)

CABA (children affected by AIDS). *See* HIV/AIDS; orphans and vulnerable children (OVC)

Cameroon, fosterage in, 139

Center for Faith-Based and Community Initiatives (USAID), 21. *See also* faith-based organizations; USAID

Cheney, Kristen, *Pillars of the Nation*, 9, 13–14, 63, 84, 88. *See also* childhood studies; children: rights and citizenship of; ethnography; youth participatory research

child circulation. *See* fosterage, of OVC; kinship
childhood studies, as subfield of anthropology, 3–
8, 31, 46–47, 49, 50, 58–59, 60–62, 133, 155, 216n1
(chap. 3). *See also* ethnography; fosterage, of
OVC; kinship; youth participatory research
children: as heads of households, 18, 29, 36, 124,
209–10, **209**; rights and citizenship of, 5, 8, 20,
25–26, 28, 29, 39, 43–57, 58–60, 71, 84, 88, 107,
127–29, 158, 170–71, 176, 186–87, 216n1 (chap.
3), 216n2 (chap. 3), 219n4. *See also* adoption;
childhood studies; ethnography; HIV/AIDS;
orphans and vulnerable children (OVC); youth
participatory research
Children Act (Uganda): of 1997, 45, 128, 162–64;
2015 amendments to, 186–87, 218n9, 219n4. *See
also* adoption: intercountry
Children in Families First (CHIFF), 161. *See also*
adoption: intercountry
child rescue, 6, 158, 164
child trafficking, 10, 95–97, 159, 161–63, 170. *See
also* adoption: intercountry; orphanages; sex
slavery
Christian Alliance for Orphans (CAFO), 159.
See also adoption: intercountry; faith-based
organizations
Christian Children's Fund, 48–49. *See also* faith-
based organizations
Clinton, Hillary Rodham, as Secretary of State, 22.
See also President's Emergency Plan for AIDS
Relief (PEPFAR)
community-based organizations (CBOs), 18, 21,
81–82. *See also* youth participatory research
condoms, 19, 20, 37, 184. *See also* abstinence education; HIV/AIDS; President's Emergency Plan
for AIDS Relief (PEPFAR); sexual education
Convention on the Rights of the Child (CRC),
26, 43–44, 45–48, 50, 59, 215n2 (chap. 2), 216n2
(chap. 3). *See also* children: rights and citizenship of; United Nations Convention on the
Rights of the Child (CRC)

Ddamulira, Faridah, 62, 64, 65–66, 67, 69, 74,
78–79, 89, 97–98, 127, 136, 149–50, 189, 191, 205,
217n5. *See also* ethnography; youth participatory research

economic policy. *See* neoliberalism; poverty
education. *See* orphans and vulnerable children
(OVC); poverty
Epstein, Helen, *The Invisible Cure*, 15, 37
Ethiopia, 161–62, 172. *See also* adoption:
intercountry
ethnography, child-centered, 2, 3, 7–9, 58–59, 60,
62, 72, 76, 78, 83–84, 106, 122, 126, 182–84, 187,
217n3 (chap. 6), 217n5. *See also* anthropology;
youth participatory research

evangelicalism. *See* faith-based organizations

faith-based organizations, 20–21, 33–34, 37–38,
174–75, 185, 216n8. *See also* abstinence education; adoption: intercountry; orphanages;
orphans and vulnerable children (OVC);
President's Emergency Plan for AIDS Relief
(PEPFAR); USAID
Fassin, Didier, 6, 31, 123, 157
fosterage, of OVC, 9–10, 28, 35, 38, 131–34, 138–39,
143, 152, 154–55, 156, 163, 166, 169, 171, 174, 176,
205, 215n2 (chap. 2). *See also* adoption: domestic; grandparents; kinship
Freud, Sigmund, *Mourning and Melancholia*, 117

generations, as social/research category, 7, 8–9, 10,
13–15, 20–23, 27, 87–88, 106, 107, 182–83, 184,
187. *See also* anthropology; childhood studies;
ethnography; youth participatory research
Geria, Martin, 63, 65, 66. *See also* African
Training, Research, and Innovation Network
(A-TRAIN); youth participatory research
Ghana, foster care in, 133. *See also* fosterage, of
OVC
Global Fund to Fight AIDS, Tuberculosis, and
Malaria, 20, 37, 183, 217n4 (chap. 6)
grandparents (*jaajas*), as guardians of orphans
and vulnerable children, 2, 21, 28–29, 36, 66, 67,
74, 91–93, 109, 111, 112–17, 120–22, 124, 125, 126,
133, 135–38, 140–41, **142**, 146–48, **149**, 153, 191–
213, **206**. *See also* fosterage, of OVC; kinship

Hague Convention on Intercountry Adoption,
161, 163, 164. *See also* adoption: intercountry
Herskovitz, Melville (American Anthropological
Association), 47. *See also* anthropology
HIV/AIDS: and adolescents, 22–23, 114, 116,
182–85, 217n7; in Africa (general), 1, 6, 8, 13,
15–22, 25–26, 28, 29–30, 35, 38, 107–8, 115, 120,
123, 131–34, 140, 151, 156, 161, 183, 184, 219n18:
in Senegal, 15; in Uganda, 7, 9, 10, 13–20, 21,
25, 35, 37–38, 51, 87, 90, 114–15, 156, 165, 182–84;
in Zimbabwe, 115, 122; children affected by
(CABA): 16, 27–28 (*see* orphans and vulnerable
children [OVC]); children's knowledge (disclosure) of status, 9, 23, 65, 107–8, 110, 113–23,
181, 182–83, 191, 203, 204, 210, 217n7; pandemic
(global), 1, 3, 9–10, 13, 15, 17–18, 21, 22, 25–26,
28, 35, 44, 108–9, 123, 126, 132, 140, 151, 156,
165, 182; and pregnancy, 13, 15, 16, 17, 19, 23, 30,
90, 109, 113, 151, 182, 183, 203: and prevention
of mother-to-child transmission (PMTCT),
13, **14**, 16, 17, 19, 22, 23, 30, 90, 182; prevention
programs, 13–15, 18–21, 23, 24, 30, 37–38, 51, 90,
114–15, 116, 119, 182–85: and abstinence education, 19–21, 23, 37–38, 116, 184–85; and sexual

education, 20–21, 183–85; sexual transmission, 15–16, 119, 183–85; testing, 13, **14**, 15, 19, 23, 79, 87, 114–15, 170, 182–83, 191, 203; treatment (*see* antiretrovirals [ARVs]). *See also* faith-based organizations; kinship: blood; orphans and vulnerable children (OVC)

humanitarianism (benevolent), 6, 9, 16, 31, 33–34, 39, 44, 158–60, 187; and children's rights, 56. *See* faith-based organizations; orphans and vulnerable children (OVC); posthumanitarianism

human rights, of children. *See* children: rights and citizenship of

Human Rights Watch, 20–21, 37. *See also* faith-based organizations

International Monetary Fund, 32

Invisible Children, 164. *See also* faith-based organizations

Joint Learning Initiative on Children and HIV/AIDS (JLICA), 126, 134, 165. *See also* HIV/AIDS

kinship, 9–10, 27, 132, 133, 134, 138, 141, 142, 148, 149, 151, 153, 154, 155, 157, 166, 167, 170, 171, 175, 191–213; and "blood" as symbol, 9–10, 131–32, 141–43, 148–51, **149**, 152, 153, 154–55, 156–57, 166–70, 173–74, 175–76, 219n5; and clan identification, 132, 137–38, 140–45, 148–52, 154, 157, 167, 169, 194, 217–18n3 (chap. 7); fictive, 152–53; and inheritance, 145, 168; maternal, 116–17, 131, 138–43, 145, 146–47, **149**, 151, 154, 155; paternal, 131–32, 136–52, 159, 167, 169: stepfathers, 139, **140**, 211, 217–18n3 (chap. 7); and patriarchal authority, 139–41, 148, 154; and witchcraft, 148–50. *See also* adoption: domestic; fosterage, of OVC; grandparents

Legal guardianship/loophole, 162–63, 186, 218n9

Mali, foster care in, 138–39. *See also* fosterage, of OVC

Mannheim, Karl, 7, 22. *See* anthropology; generations, as social/research category

maternal/matrilineal kin. *See* kinship

Millennium Declaration (UN), 29. *See also* UN Millenium Declaration

Millennium Development Goals (MDG) (UNICEF), 22, 30, 215n2 (chap. 1). *See also* UNICEF

MTV Staying Alive Foundation, 183. *See also* HIV/AIDS: and adolescents

Mugumya, Herbert, 30–31. *See also* USAID

Museveni, Janet, as First Lady of Uganda, 35. *See also* Uganda Women's Effort to Save Orphans

Museveni, Yoweri, as president of Uganda, 32–33, 37–38, 93, 186. *See also* Children Act; HIV/AIDS: in Uganda

neocolonialism, 24, 38, 52. *See also* anthropology; neoliberalism

neoliberalism, 5, 21, 31–34, 39, 43–44, 50, 87, 97. *See also* nongovernmental organizations (NGOs); poverty

nongovernmental organizations (NGOs), 16, 18, 20, 21–22, 25, 27–28, 32–37, 44, 48–49, 50, 52, 54–55, 60, 62, 77, 78, 109, 186, 219n14. *See also* children: rights and citizenship of; faith-based organizations; orphans and vulnerable children (OVC)

Nyombi, Peter, 164, 186, 218n9. *See also* Children Act; Museveni, Yoweri

Obama, Barack, administration, 22, 183. *See also* President's Emergency Plan for AIDS Relief (PEPFAR).

Okiror, John, 26, 31

147 Million Orphans, 159–60. *See also* faith-based organizations

Opolot, Simon, 63, **64**, 66, 67–68. *See also* African Training, Research, and Innovation Network (A-TRAIN); youth participatory research

orphanages, 10, 38, 135, 157–66, 167, 172, 174–75, 181, 185, 186, 218n10, 218n13, 218n15; in Europe, 158. *See also* adoption; alternative care; orphan industrial complex; orphans and vulnerable children (OVC)

orphan industrial complex, 10, 159, 160–61, 164, 186. *See also* adoption; orphanages; orphans and vulnerable children (OVC)

orphans and vulnerable children (OVC): caused by war, 29, 35, 109, 158–59, 161, 164–65, 195; in context of extended families and local communities, 2, 7, 16, 18, 21, 25, 26–27, 35, 38, 44, 47, 49, 60, 76–77, 84, 111, 116, 121–22, 137, 155, 158, 166, 172, 185, 191–213; definitions of, 2–3, 7, 16–17, 24–25, 26–27, **28**, 29–30, 31, 33–35, 36–37, 38, 39, 44, 47, 49–50, 51–52, 60, 83, 158, 181, 185, 187, 217n8; double orphans, 88, 91, 93, 101, 104, **125**, 198–99; institutionalization of (*see* orphanages); local terms for: *balekwa* (Luganda), 118, 217n8; *ekokit* (Ateso), 26–27; *enfunzi* (Luganda), 26; *mulekwa* (Luganda), 26, 36, 118, 192, 195, 198, 211, 217n8; "orphan addiction," 10, **28**, 174, 185; "orphan crisis," 8, 9, 16, 18, 25, 27, **28**, 31, 34–35, 153, 156, 159–60, 165, 174, 185; orphan tourism, 160; self-identification of children as, 1, 24, 36, 38–39, 48–49, 57, 61, 82–83, 118, 142–43, 196; statistics: in Sub-Saharan Africa, 16, 18, 26; in Uganda, 18, 25, 26, 28–31, 50–51, 53–54, 60, 215n1 (Intro.). *See also* adoption; alternative care; children: rights

orphans and vulnerable children (OVC)
(*continued*)
and citizenship of; faith-based organizations;
fosterage, of OVC; HIV/AIDS; kinship; orphanages; orphan industrial complex; poverty;
youth participatory research
Oulanyah, Dorothy (UNICEF), 24, 27, 29–30, 36,
51, 53. *See also* UNICEF

Parsons, Ross, 115, 122
paternal/patrilineal kin. *See* kinship
PEPFAR. *See* President's Emergency Plan for
AIDS Relief
PEPFAR Watch, 20. *See also* abstinence education;
condoms; President's Emergency Plan for
AIDS Relief (PEPFAR)
posthumanitarianism, 6–7
poverty: and aid resources, 3, 32–33, 34, 56, 105;
and child abandonment, 158, 163–66, 171–72;
and children as "deserving poor," 6, 33, 39, 50,
134; education as solution to, 5, 35, 78, 99, 101–
4, 123; and female-headed households, 141, 154;
of orphans and vulnerable children (OVC), 2,
5–6, 9, 18, 27–28, 29, 32–35, 37, 39, 44, 53, 56, 84,
87–88, 98, 100–104, 105, 108, 118, 123, 126, 132,
134, 136, 138, 141, 145, 154–55, 158, 160, 162, 163,
165–66, 171–72, 176. *See also* adoption; fosterage, of OVC; kinship; orphans and vulnerable
children (OVC); youth participatory research
Presidential Advisory Council on HIV/AIDS
(United States), 19
President's Emergency Plan for AIDS Relief
(PEPFAR), 14, 18–23, 33–34, 37, 116, 183, 185,
217n4 (chap. 6). *See also* abstinence education;
condoms; faith-based organizations; HIV/
AIDS: prevention programs
prostitution, 21. *See also* President's Emergency
Plan for AIDS Relief (PEPFAR); sexual
education
Protecting the Vulnerable (PTV), 29–30. *See also*
UNICEF

Ranger, Terence, Evangelical Christianity and
Democracy in Africa, 33
Rapid Assessment, Analysis, and Action Planning
(RAAAP), 18. *See also* USAID
Riley, Mark, 159, 162, 164, 165, 172–73, 174–75. *See
also* adoption: alternative care models; alterna-
tive care; fosterage, of OVC; orphanages

Save the Children, 43, 53, 56, 60
Seeley, Janet, *HIV and East Africa*, 15–16
Senegal, HIV/AIDS in, 15
sex slavery (and sex trafficking), 95–97, 170, 174.
See also child trafficking

sexual education, 20–21, 183–85. *See also*
abstinence education; condoms; faith-based
organizations; HIV/AIDS
sexual network theory (Thornton), 15–16
structural adjustment program (SAP), 32. *See also*
poverty

Thornton, Robert, *Unimagined Community*,
15, 184

Uganda AIDS Commission, 17, 21, 114, 182. *See
also* HIV/AIDS: in Uganda
Uganda Center for Accountability, 37
Uganda Children Act. *See* Children Act
Uganda Child Rights NGO Network (UCRNN),
52, 54–55, 219n4. *See also* children: rights and
citizenship of; Children Act
Uganda Ministry of Gender, Labour, and Social
Development, 29, 30, 54, 165, 186
Uganda OVC National Implementation Unit,
26–27, 53, 60. *See also* orphans and vulnerable
children (OVC)
Uganda Women's Effort to Save Orphans
(UWESO), 35–36, 38, 57, 109
UNAIDS (Joint United Nations Programme on
HIV/AIDS), 18, 23, 26, 183–84
UNFPA (United Nations Population Fund;
originally United Nations Fund for Population
Activities), 34, 183
UNICEF (United Nations Children's Fund; origi-
nally United Nations International Children's
Emergency Fund), 8, 16, 17, 18, 21, 23, 24, 26–27,
29–30, 36, 45–46, 47–48, 51, 53, 54–55, 135, 159,
161, 176, 181, 182–83, 217n8. *See also* children:
rights and citizenship of; orphans and vulner-
able children (OVC)
United Nations (UN). *See* UNICEF
United Nations Children's Fund. *See* UNICEF;
United Nations Convention on the Rights of
the Child (CRC)
United Nations Convention on the Rights of the
Child (CRC), 26, 43–48, 50, 59, 215n2 (chap. 2),
216n3 (chap. 3). *See also* children: rights and
citizenship of
Universal Declaration of Human Rights, 45, 47.
See also anthropology; children: rights and
citizenship of
UN Millennium Declaration, 29
USAID (United States Agency for International
Development), 18, 21, 30–31
UWESO. *See* Uganda Women's Effort to Save
Orphans

Viva International, 21, 39, 48. *See also* nongovernmental organizations (NGOs)

voluntary counseling and testing (VCT). *See* HIV/
   AIDS: testing

Waiswa, Baker, 35, 109. *See also* Uganda Women's
   Effort to Save Orphans (UWESO)
Webb, Douglas, 22
Whyte, Susan. R., *Second Chances*, 13–15, 20
women's studies, 3, 4
World Bank, 17, 32, 44, 102, 217n4 (chap. 6)
World Food Programme, 18
World Health Organization (WHO), 217n7

Young Lives Project, 5. *See also* poverty
youth participatory research, 6, 8, 10, 14, 45, 49,
   53, 58–84, 107, 185; and youth research assistants (RAs), 7–9, 13, 58–84, **64, 67, 68, 70, 71,
   80**, 148, 150, 152, 153, 181, 182, 187, 191–213. *See
   also* anthropology; children: rights and citizenship of; ethnography; orphans and vulnerable
   children (OVC)

Zimbabwe, and children with HIV/AIDS,
   115, 122

www.ingramcontent.com/pod-product-compliance
Lightning Source LLC
Chambersburg PA
CBHW032130020426
42334CB00016B/1099